EMERIL LAGASSE FRENCH DOOR LARGE

Air Fryer Oven Cookbook

1500 Days Delicious Recipes to Elevate practically any meal, customized for your party, including Everyday Side Dishes, Snacks, Desserts & More

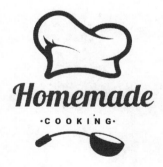

Homemade

·COOKING·

Holly R. Ahmed

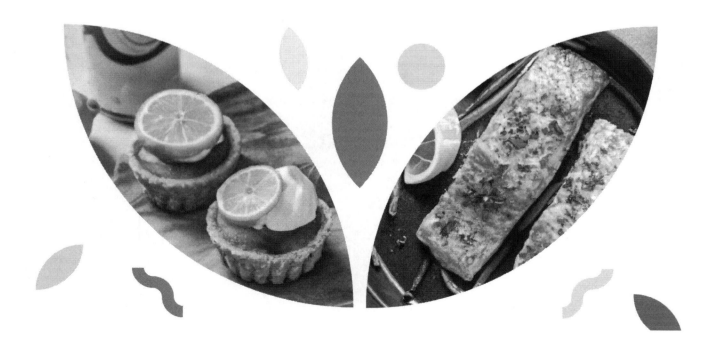

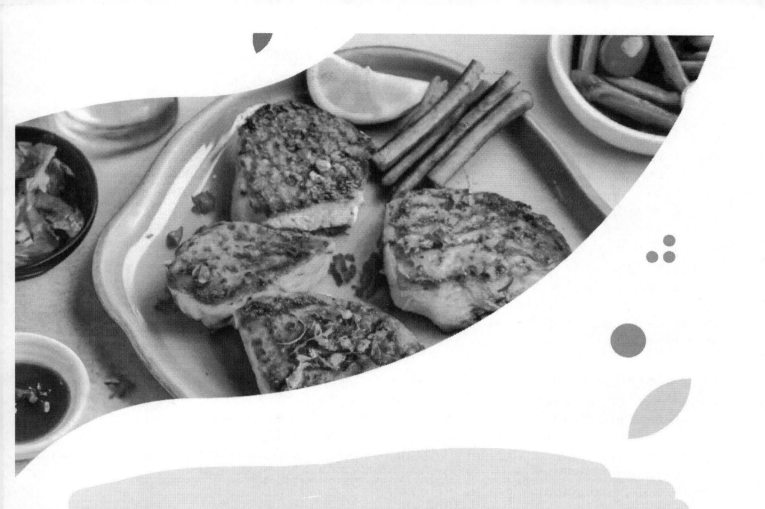

CONTENTS

INTRODUCTION   4

Bread And Breakfast Recipes   7

Appetizers And Snacks Recipes
17

Beef ,pork & Lamb Recipes   28

Poultry Recipes   39

Vegetable Side Dishes Recipes 50

Vegetarians Recipes 60

Sandwiches And Burgers Recipes
71

Fish And Seafood Recipes   84

Desserts And Sweets Recipes   94

Shopping List 104

APPENDIX A: Measurement
Conversions   105

Appendix B : Recipes Index   107

INTRODUCTION

Hello, everyone. I'm Holly R. Ahmed, and I'm absolutely delighted to introduce you to my latest culinary adventure, the "Emeril Lagasse Pressure Air Fryer Cookbook." As a passionate home cook with a knack for creating mouthwatering meals and a busy professional with limited time to spare, I understand the importance of cooking that's not only delicious but also convenient. That's precisely why I embarked on this journey to craft a cookbook specifically tailored to the incredible Emeril Lagasse Pressure Air Fryer.

With a background in culinary arts and a deep love for cooking that has been passed down through generations, I've had the privilege of experimenting with countless kitchen gadgets and techniques. The Emeril Lagasse Pressure Air Fryer immediately caught my attention with its ability to combine pressure cooking and air frying, offering the best of both worlds. It became my trusted kitchen companion, saving me time and energy without compromising on flavor and texture.

The purpose of this cookbook is simple yet profound—to empower home cooks of all levels to make the most of their Emeril Lagasse Pressure Air Fryer. Inside these pages, you'll find a treasure trove of delectable recipes, each meticulously crafted and tested to ensure foolproof results. Whether you're a seasoned cook looking to expand your culinary horizons or a beginner taking your first steps in the kitchen, I've included detailed step-by-step instructions, comprehensive shopping lists, precise cooking times, and a plethora of practical cooking tips to guide you every step of the way.

From savory stews that melt in your mouth to crispy delights that tantalize your taste buds, this cookbook covers it all. I've poured my heart and soul into these recipes, aiming to make your cooking experience both enjoyable and hassle-free. With the Emeril Lagasse Pressure Air Fryer at your side and this cookbook as your trusty guide, you'll be able to whip up restaurant-quality dishes that will impress family and friends alike.

So, join me on this culinary journey, and let's embrace the convenience and deliciousness that the Emeril Lagasse Pressure Air Fryer brings to our kitchens. Whether you're seeking weekday dinner solutions or weekend indulgences, this cookbook is here to inspire and simplify your cooking experience, one delectable recipe at a time. Cheers to flavor-packed meals and unforgettable moments shared around the table!

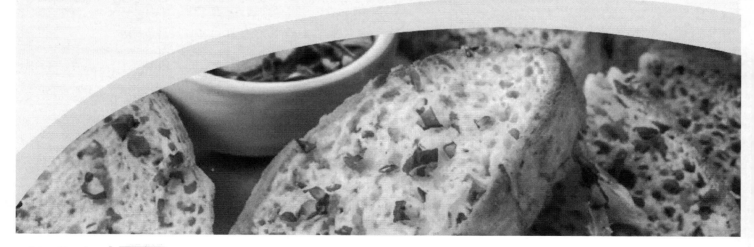

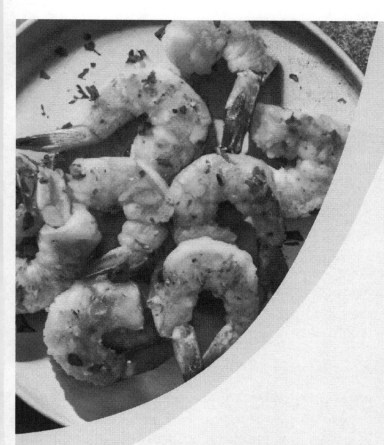

THE EMERIL LAGASSE 26 QT EXTRA LARGE AIR FRYER OFFERS A VARIETY OF COOKING METHODS

Air Fry: The primary cooking method of the air fryer, which uses powerful hot air circulation to crisp and brown food without the need for excessive oil. It's perfect for making crispy fries, chicken wings, and other traditionally fried foods with less fat.

Roast: The air fryer can roast meats, vegetables, and even whole chickens to perfection, ensuring a tender and juicy interior with a flavorful, crispy exterior.

Bake: You can use the air fryer for baking purposes, making it suitable for preparing everything from cakes and muffins to cookies and bread.

Grill: Many air fryer models, including the Emeril Lagasse 26 QT, come with grilling accessories that allow you to achieve grill-like results for steaks, burgers, and even kebabs.

Dehydrate: With its low-temperature settings, the air fryer can dehydrate fruits, vegetables, and herbs, creating homemade dried snacks and ingredients for recipes.

Reheat: The air fryer is excellent for reheating leftovers, as it can restore their crispiness and freshness, unlike a microwave.

Rotisserie Cook: The Emeril Lagasse 26 QT Extra Large Air Fryer often comes with a rotisserie function, enabling you to roast whole chickens or other meats on a rotating spit, ensuring even cooking and succulent results.

Broil: By using the air fryer's top heating element, you can achieve a broiled finish on dishes like casseroles and gratins.

GETTING TO KNOW EMERIL LAGASSE 26 QT EXTRA LARGE AIR FRYER

The Emeril Lagasse 26 QT Extra Large Air Fryer is a kitchen appliance that combines versatility and capacity. With its spacious 26-quart interior, this air fryer allows for ample cooking space, making it ideal for preparing large meals and accommodating a variety of dishes. Equipped with advanced air frying technology, it provides a healthier cooking alternative by crisping and browning food with little to no oil, resulting in deliciously crispy and golden textures. Emeril Lagasse's signature appliance features user-friendly controls, multiple cooking presets, and precise temperature settings, making it suitable for a wide range of cooking applications, from frying and roasting to baking and dehydrating. This air fryer is a go-to choice for those seeking convenience and versatility in their kitchen, delivering mouthwatering meals with ease.

THE EMERIL LAGASSE 26 QT EXTRA LARGE AIR FRYER BRINGS YOU THE BENEFITS OF COOKING IN THE KITCHEN

GENEROUS CAPACITY

This air fryer's extra-large 26-quart capacity allows you to cook larger portions, making it suitable for family meals and gatherings. It's an ideal choice when you need to prepare ample food without overcrowding the cooking space.

HEALTHIER COOKING

The air fryer uses powerful hot air circulation to achieve crispy textures with minimal oil. It significantly reduces the fat content in your dishes, promoting healthier eating habits without compromising on taste.

VERSATILE COOKING METHODS

From air frying for crispy results to roasting for tender meats, baking for delicious pastries, grilling for BBQ-like flavors, dehydrating for homemade snacks, and more, this appliance accommodates a wide range of cooking techniques to suit various recipes.

EASE OF USE

Featuring user-friendly controls and pre-programmed cooking presets, the Emeril Lagasse Air Fryer is easy to operate. Whether you're a beginner or a seasoned cook, you can quickly adapt to its functions and prepare meals with confidence.

PRECISE TEMPERATURE CONTROL

The air fryer offers precise temperature settings, allowing you to fine-tune the cooking process. This precision ensures that your dishes come out perfectly cooked and tailored to your preferences.

TIME-SAVING

With rapid hot air circulation, the air fryer typically cooks food faster than traditional methods. It's a time-efficient option for busy individuals and families, helping you get meals on the table quicker.

EASY CLEANUP

Many parts of the air fryer are designed to be non-stick and removable, making cleanup hassle-free. These components are often dishwasher-safe, simplifying the post-cooking maintenance.

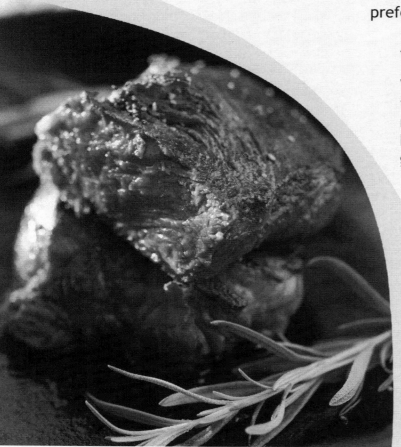

Bread And Breakfast Recipes

Mashed Potato Taquitos With Hot Sauce 8
Viking Toast..8
Green Onion Pancakes..8
Blueberry French Toast Sticks 9
Morning Potato Cakes 9
Meaty Omelet..9
Morning Loaded Potato Skins..9
Maple-peach And Apple Oatmeal 10
Baked Eggs...10
Blueberry Muffins 10
Lorraine Egg Cups 11
Eggless Mung Bean Tart..11
Breakfast Frittata...11
Crispy Samosa Rolls..11
Nordic Salmon Quiche 12
Apple-cinnamon-walnut Muffins......................................12
Garlic Bread Knots...12
Avocado Toasts With Poached Eggs 13
Parsley Egg Scramble With Cottage Cheese 13
Pizza Dough...13
Spring Vegetable Omelet 14
Green Egg Quiche 14
Coffee Cake 14
Roasted Vegetable Frittata 15
Fried Pb&j 15
Buttermilk Biscuits...16
Sweet And Spicy Pumpkin Scones 16

BREAD AND BREAKFAST RECIPES

Mashed Potato Taquitos With Hot Sauce

Servings: 4
Cooking Time: 30 Minutes

Ingredients:
- 1 potato, peeled and cubed
- 2 tbsp milk
- 2 garlic cloves, minced
- Salt and pepper to taste
- ½ tsp ground cumin
- 2 tbsp minced scallions
- 4 corn tortillas
- 1 cup red chili sauce
- 1 avocado, sliced
- 2 tbsp cilantro, chopped

Directions:
1. In a pot fitted with a steamer basket, cook the potato cubes for 15 minutes on the stovetop. Pour the potato cubes into a bowl and mash with a potato masher. Add the milk, garlic, salt, pepper, and cumin and stir. Add the scallions and cilantro and stir them into the mixture.
2. Preheat air fryer to 390°F. Run the tortillas under water for a second, then place them in the greased frying basket. Air Fry for 1 minute. Lay the tortillas on a flat surface. Place an equal amount of the potato filling in the center of each. Roll the tortilla sides over the filling and place seam-side down in the frying basket. Fry for 7 minutes or until the tortillas are golden and slightly crisp. Serve with chili sauce and avocado slices. Enjoy!

Viking Toast

Servings: 2
Cooking Time: 20 Minutes

Ingredients:
- 2 tbsp minced green chili pepper
- 1 avocado, pressed
- 1 clove garlic, minced
- ¼ tsp lemon juice
- Salt and pepper to taste
- 2 bread slices
- 2 plum tomatoes, sliced
- 4 oz smoked salmon
- ¼ diced peeled red onion

Directions:
1. Preheat air fryer at 350°F. Combine the avocado, garlic, lemon juice, and salt in a bowl until you reach your desired consistency. Spread avocado mixture on the bread slices.
2. Top with tomato slices and sprinkle with black pepper. Place bread slices in the frying basket and Bake for 5 minutes. Transfer to a plate. Top each bread slice with salmon, green chili pepper, and red onion. Serve.

Green Onion Pancakes

Servings: 4
Cooking Time: 8 Minutes

Ingredients:
- 2 cup all-purpose flour
- ½ teaspoon salt
- ¾ cup hot water
- 1 tablespoon vegetable oil
- 1 tablespoon butter, melted
- 2 cups finely chopped green onions
- 1 tablespoon black sesame seeds, for garnish

Directions:
1. In a large bowl, whisk together the flour and salt. Make a well in the center and pour in the hot water. Quickly stir the flour mixture together until a dough forms. Knead the dough for 5 minutes; then cover with a warm, wet towel and set aside for 30 minutes to rest.
2. In a small bowl, mix together the vegetable oil and melted butter.
3. On a floured surface, place the dough and cut it into 8 pieces. Working with 1 piece of dough at a time, use a rolling pin to roll out the dough until it's ¼ inch thick; then brush the surface with the oil and butter mixture and sprinkle with green onions. Next, fold the dough in half and

then in half again. Roll out the dough again until it's ¼ inch thick and brush with the oil and butter mixture and green onions. Fold the dough in half and then in half again and roll out one last time until it's ¼ inch thick. Repeat this technique with all 8 pieces.

4. Meanwhile, preheat the air fryer to 400°F.

5. Place 1 or 2 pancakes into the air fryer basket (or as many as will fit in your fryer), and cook for 2 minutes or until crispy and golden brown. Repeat until all the pancakes are cooked. Top with black sesame seeds for garnish, if desired.

Blueberry French Toast Sticks

Servings: 4
Cooking Time: 20 Minutes

Ingredients:
- 3 bread slices, cut into strips
- 1 tbsp butter, melted
- 2 eggs
- 1 tbsp milk
- 1 tbsp sugar
- ½ tsp vanilla extract
- 1 cup fresh blueberries
- 1 tbsp lemon juice

Directions:
1. Preheat air fryer to 380°F. After laying the bread strips on a plate, sprinkle some melted butter over each piece. Whisk the eggs, milk, vanilla, and sugar, then dip the bread in the mix. Place on a wire rack to let the batter drip. Put the bread strips in the air fryer and Air Fry for 5-7 minutes. Use tongs to flip them once and cook until golden. With a fork, smash the blueberries and lemon juice together. Spoon the blueberries sauce over the French sticks. Serve immediately.

Morning Potato Cakes

Servings: 6
Cooking Time: 50 Minutes

Ingredients:
- 4 Yukon Gold potatoes
- 2 cups kale, chopped
- 1 cup rice flour
- ¼ cup cornstarch
- ¾ cup milk
- 2 tbsp lemon juice
- 2 tsp dried rosemary
- 2 tsp shallot powder
- Salt and pepper to taste
- ½ tsp turmeric powder

Directions:
1. Preheat air fryer to 390°F. Scrub the potatoes and put them in the air fryer. Bake for 30 minutes or until soft. When cool, chop them into small pieces and place them in a bowl. Mash with a potato masher or fork. Add kale, rice flour, cornstarch, milk, lemon juice, rosemary, shallot powder, salt, pepper, and turmeric. Stir well.

2. Make 12 balls out of the mixture and smash them lightly with your hands to make patties. Place them in the greased frying basket, and Air Fry for 10-12 minutes, flipping once, until golden and cooked through. Serve.

Meaty Omelet

Servings: 4
Cooking Time: 20 Minutes

Ingredients:
- 6 eggs
- ½ cup grated Swiss cheese
- 3 breakfast sausages, sliced
- 8 bacon strips, sliced
- Salt and pepper to taste

Directions:
1. Preheat air fryer to 360°F. In a bowl, beat the eggs and stir in Swiss cheese, sausages and bacon. Transfer the mixture to a baking dish and set in the fryer. Bake for 15 minutes or until golden and crisp. Season and serve.

Morning Loaded Potato Skins

Servings: 4
Cooking Time: 55 Minutes

Ingredients:
- 2 large potatoes
- 1 fried bacon slice, chopped
- Salt and pepper to taste
- 1 tbsp chopped dill
- 1 ½ tbsp butter
- 2 tbsp milk
- 4 eggs
- 1 scallion, sliced

- ¼ cup grated fontina cheese
- 2 tbsp chopped parsley

Directions:

1. Preheat air fryer to 400°F. Wash each potato and poke with fork 3 or 4 times. Place in the frying basket and bake for 40-45 minutes. Remove the potatoes and let cool until they can be handled. Cut each potato in half lengthwise. Scoop out potato flesh but leave enough to maintain the structure of the potato. Transfer the potato flesh to a medium bowl and stir in salt, pepper, dill, bacon, butter, and milk until mashed with some chunky pieces.

2. Fill the potato skin halves with the potato mixture and press the center of the filling with a spoon about ½-inch deep. Crack an egg in the center of each potato, then top with scallions and cheese. Return the potatoes to the air fryer and bake for 3 to 5 minutes until the egg is cooked to preferred doneness and cheese is melted. Serve immediately sprinkled with parsley.

Maple-peach And Apple Oatmeal

Servings: 4
Cooking Time: 15 Minutes

Ingredients:

- 2 cups old-fashioned rolled oats
- ½ tsp baking powder
- 1 ½ tsp ground cinnamon
- ¼ tsp ground flaxseeds
- ⅛ tsp salt
- 1 ¼ cups vanilla almond milk
- ¼ cup maple syrup
- 1 tsp vanilla extract
- 1 peeled peach, diced
- 1 peeled apple, diced

Directions:

1. Preheat air fryer to 350°F. Mix oats, baking powder, cinnamon, flaxseed, and salt in a large bowl. Next, stir in almond milk, maple syrup, vanilla, and ¾ of the diced peaches, and ¾ of the diced apple. Grease 6 ramekins. Divide the batter evenly between the ramekins and transfer the ramekins to the frying basket. Bake in the air fryer for 8-10 minutes until the top is golden and set. Garnish with the rest of the peaches and apples. Serve.

Baked Eggs

Servings: 4
Cooking Time: 6 Minutes

Ingredients:

- 4 large eggs
- ⅛ teaspoon black pepper
- ⅛ teaspoon salt

Directions:

1. Preheat the air fryer to 330°F. Place 4 silicone muffin liners into the air fryer basket.
2. Crack 1 egg at a time into each silicone muffin liner. Sprinkle with black pepper and salt.
3. Bake for 6 minutes. Remove and let cool 2 minutes prior to serving.

Blueberry Muffins

Servings: 8
Cooking Time: 14 Minutes

Ingredients:

- 1⅓ cups flour
- ½ cup sugar
- 2 teaspoons baking powder
- ¼ teaspoon salt
- ⅓ cup canola oil
- 1 egg
- ½ cup milk
- ⅔ cup blueberries, fresh or frozen and thawed
- 8 foil muffin cups including paper liners

Directions:

1. Preheat air fryer to 330°F.
2. In a medium bowl, stir together flour, sugar, baking powder, and salt.
3. In a separate bowl, combine oil, egg, and milk and mix well.
4. Add egg mixture to dry ingredients and stir just until moistened.
5. Gently stir in blueberries.
6. Spoon batter evenly into muffin cups.
7. Place 4 muffin cups in air fryer basket and bake at 330°F for 14 minutes or until tops spring back when touched lightly.
8. Repeat previous step to cook remaining muffins.

Lorraine Egg Cups

Servings: 6
Cooking Time: 30 Minutes

Ingredients:
- 3 eggs
- 2 tbsp half-and-half
- Garlic salt and pepper to taste
- 2 tbsp diced white onion
- 1 tbs dried parsley
- 3 oz cooked bacon, crumbled
- ¼ cup grated Swiss cheese
- 1 tomato, sliced

Directions:
1. Preheat air fryer at 350°F. Whisk the egg, half-and-half, garlic sea salt, parsley and black pepper in a bowl. Divide onion, bacon, and cheese between 6 lightly greased silicone cupcakes. Spread the egg mixture between cupcakes evenly. Top each cup with 1 tomato slice. Place them in the frying basket and Bake for 8-10 minutes. Serve immediately.

Eggless Mung Bean Tart

Servings: 2
Cooking Time: 20 Minutes

Ingredients:
- 2 tsp soy sauce
- 1 tsp lime juice
- 1 large garlic clove, minced or pressed
- ½ tsp red chili flakes
- ½ cup mung beans, soaked
- Salt and pepper to taste
- ½ minced shallot
- 1 green onion, chopped

Directions:
1. Preheat the air fryer to 390°F. Add the soy sauce, lime juice, garlic, and chili flakes to a bowl and stir. Set aside. Place the drained beans in a blender along with ½ cup of water, salt, and pepper. Blend until smooth. Stir in shallot and green onion, but do not blend.
2. Pour the batter into a greased baking pan. Bake for 15 minutes in the air fryer until golden. A knife inserted in the center should come out clean. Once cooked, cut the "quiche" into quarters. Drizzle with sauce and serve.

Breakfast Frittata

Servings:2
Cooking Time: 25 Minutes

Ingredients:
- 4 cooked pancetta slices, chopped
- 5 eggs
- Salt and pepper to taste
- ½ leek, thinly sliced
- ½ cup grated cheddar cheese
- 1 tomato, sliced
- 1 cup iceberg lettuce, torn
- 2 tbsp milk

Directions:
1. Preheat air fryer to 320°F. Beat the eggs, milk, salt, and pepper in a bowl. Mix in pancetta and cheddar. Transfer to a greased with olive oil baking pan. Top with tomato slices and leek and place it in the frying basket. Bake for 14 minutes. Let cool for 5 minutes. Serve with lettuce.

Crispy Samosa Rolls

Servings: 4
Cooking Time: 30 Minutes

Ingredients:
- 2/3 cup canned peas
- 4 scallions, finely sliced
- 2 cups grated potatoes
- 2 tbsp lemon juice
- 1 tsp ground ginger
- 1 tsp curry powder
- 1 tsp Garam masala
- ¼ cup chickpea flour
- 1 tbsp tahini
- 8 rice paper wrappers

Directions:
1. Preheat air fryer to 350°F. Mix the peas, scallions, potatoes, lemon juice, ginger, curry powder, Garam masala, and chickpea flour in a bowl. In another bowl, whisk tahini and 1/3 cup of water until combined. Set aside on a plate.
2. Submerge the rice wrappers, one by one, into the tahini mixture until they begin to soften and set aside on a plate.
3. Fill each wrap with 1/3 cup of the veggie mixture and wrap them into a roll. Bake for 15 minutes until golden brown and crispy, turning once. Serve right away.

Nordic Salmon Quiche

Servings: 4
Cooking Time: 30 Minutes

Ingredients:
- ¼ cup shredded mozzarella cheese
- ¼ cup shredded Gruyere cheese
- 1 refrigerated pie crust
- 2 eggs
- ¼ cup milk
- Salt and pepper to taste
- 1 tsp dry dill
- 5 oz cooked salmon
- 1 large tomato, diced

Directions:
1. Preheat air fryer to 360°F. In a baking dish, add the crust and press firmly. Trim off any excess edges. Poke a few holes. Beat the eggs in a bowl. Stir in the milk, dill, tomato, salmon, half of the cheeses, salt, and pepper. Mix well as break the salmon into chunks, mixing it evenly among other ingredients. Transfer the mix to the baking dish.
2. Bake in the fryer for 15 minutes until firm and almost crusty. Slide the basket out and top with the remaining cheeses. Cook further for 5 minutes, or until golden brown. Let cool slightly and serve.

Apple-cinnamon-walnut Muffins

Servings: 8
Cooking Time: 11 Minutes

Ingredients:
- 1 cup flour
- ⅓ cup sugar
- 1 teaspoon baking powder
- ¼ teaspoon baking soda
- ¼ teaspoon salt
- 1 teaspoon cinnamon
- ¼ teaspoon ginger
- ¼ teaspoon nutmeg
- 1 egg
- 2 tablespoons pancake syrup, plus 2 teaspoons
- 2 tablespoons melted butter, plus 2 teaspoons
- ¾ cup unsweetened applesauce
- ½ teaspoon vanilla extract
- ¼ cup chopped walnuts
- ¼ cup diced apple
- 8 foil muffin cups, liners removed and sprayed with cooking spray

Directions:
1. Preheat air fryer to 330°F.
2. In a large bowl, stir together flour, sugar, baking powder, baking soda, salt, cinnamon, ginger, and nutmeg.
3. In a small bowl, beat egg until frothy. Add syrup, butter, applesauce, and vanilla and mix well.
4. Pour egg mixture into dry ingredients and stir just until moistened.
5. Gently stir in nuts and diced apple.
6. Divide batter among the 8 muffin cups.
7. Place 4 muffin cups in air fryer basket and cook at 330°F for 11minutes.
8. Repeat with remaining 4 muffins or until toothpick inserted in center comes out clean.

Garlic Bread Knots

Servings: 8
Cooking Time: 5 Minutes

Ingredients:
- ¼ cup melted butter
- 2 teaspoons garlic powder
- 1 teaspoon dried parsley
- 1 (11-ounce) tube of refrigerated French bread dough

Directions:
1. Mix the melted butter, garlic powder and dried parsley in a small bowl and set it aside.
2. To make smaller knots, cut the long tube of bread dough into 16 slices. If you want to make bigger knots, slice the dough into 8 slices. Shape each slice into a long rope about 6 inches long by rolling it on a flat surface with the palm of your hands. Tie each rope into a knot and place them on a plate.
3. Preheat the air fryer to 350°F.
4. Transfer half of the bread knots into the air fryer basket, leaving space in between each knot. Brush each knot with the butter mixture using a pastry brush.
5. Air-fry for 5 minutes. Remove the baked knots and brush a little more of the garlic butter mixture on each. Repeat with the remaining bread knots and serve warm.

Avocado Toasts With Poached Eggs

Servings: 4
Cooking Time: 15 Minutes

Ingredients:
- 4 eggs
- Salt and pepper to taste
- 4 bread pieces, toasted
- 1 pitted avocado, sliced
- ½ tsp chili powder
- ½ tsp dried rosemary

Directions:
1. Preheat air fryer to 320°F. Crack 1 egg into each greased ramekin and season with salt and black pepper. Place the ramekins into the air frying basket. Bake for 6-8 minutes.
2. Scoop the flesh of the avocado into a small bowl. Season with salt, black pepper, chili powderp and rosemary. Using a fork, smash the avocado lightly. Spread the smashed avocado evenly over toasted bread slices. Remove the eggs from the air fryer and gently spoon one onto each slice of avocado toast. Serve and enjoy!

Parsley Egg Scramble With Cottage Cheese

Servings:2
Cooking Time: 15 Minutes

Ingredients:
- 1 tbsp cottage cheese, crumbled
- 4 eggs
- Salt and pepper to taste
- 2 tsp heavy cream
- 1 tbsp chopped parsley

Directions:
1. Preheat air fryer to 400°F. Grease a baking pan with olive oil. Beat the eggs, salt, and pepper in a bowl. Pour it into the pan, place the pan in the frying basket, and Air Fry for 5 minutes. Using a silicone spatula, stir in heavy cream, cottage cheese, and half of parsley and Air Fry for another 2 minutes. Scatter with parsley to serve.

Pizza Dough

Servings: 3
Cooking Time: 10 Minutes

Ingredients:
- 4 cups bread flour, pizza ("00") flour or all-purpose flour
- 1 teaspoon active dry yeast
- 2 teaspoons sugar
- 2 teaspoons salt
- 1½ cups water
- 1 tablespoon olive oil

Directions:
1. Combine the flour, yeast, sugar and salt in the bowl of a stand mixer. Add the olive oil to the flour mixture and start to mix using the dough hook attachment. As you're mixing, add 1¼ cups of the water, mixing until the dough comes together. Continue to knead the dough with the dough hook for another 10 minutes, adding enough water to the dough to get it to the right consistency.
2. Transfer the dough to a floured counter and divide it into 3 equal portions. Roll each portion into a ball. Lightly coat each dough ball with oil and transfer to the refrigerator, covered with plastic wrap. You can place them all on a baking sheet, or place each dough ball into its own oiled zipper sealable plastic bag or container. (You can freeze the dough balls at this stage, removing as much air as possible from the oiled bag.) Keep in the refrigerator for at least one day, or as long as five days.
3. When you're ready to use the dough, remove your dough from the refrigerator at least 1 hour prior to baking and let it sit on the counter, covered gently with plastic wrap.

Spring Vegetable Omelet

Servings: 4
Cooking Time: 20 Minutes

Ingredients:
- ¼ cup chopped broccoli, lightly steamed
- ½ cup grated cheddar cheese
- 6 eggs
- ¼ cup steamed kale
- 1 green onion, chopped
- Salt and pepper to taste

Directions:
1. Preheat air fryer to 360°F. In a bowl, beat the eggs. Stir in kale, broccoli, green onion, and cheddar cheese. Transfer the mixture to a greased baking dish and Bake in the fryer for 15 minutes until golden and crisp. Season to taste and serve immediately.

Green Egg Quiche

Servings: 4
Cooking Time: 30 Minutes

Ingredients:
- 1 cup broccoli florets
- 2 cups baby spinach
- 2 garlic cloves, minced
- ¼ tsp ground nutmeg
- 1 tbsp olive oil
- Salt and pepper to taste
- 4 eggs
- 2 scallions, chopped
- 1 red onion, chopped
- 1 tbsp sour cream
- ½ cup grated fontina cheese

Directions:
1. Preheat air fryer to 375°F. Combine broccoli, spinach, onion, garlic, nutmeg, olive oil, and salt in a medium bowl, tossing to coat. Arrange the broccoli in a single layer in the parchment-lined frying basket and cook for 5 minutes. Remove and set to the side.
2. Use the same medium bowl to whisk eggs, salt, pepper, scallions, and sour cream. Add the roasted broccoli and ¼ cup fontina cheese until all ingredients are well combined. Pour the mixture into a greased baking dish and top with cheese. Bake in the air fryer for 15-18 minutes until the center is set. Serve and enjoy.

Coffee Cake

Servings: 8
Cooking Time: 35 Minutes

Ingredients:
- 4 tablespoons butter, melted and divided
- ⅓ cup cane sugar
- ¼ cup brown sugar
- 1 large egg
- 1 cup plus 6 teaspoons milk, divided
- 1 teaspoon vanilla extract
- 2 cups all-purpose flour
- 1½ teaspoons baking powder
- ¼ teaspoon salt
- 2 teaspoons ground cinnamon
- ⅓ cup chopped pecans
- ⅓ cup powdered sugar

Directions:
1. Preheat the air fryer to 325°F.
2. Using a hand mixer or stand mixer, in a medium bowl, cream together the butter, cane sugar, brown sugar, the egg, 1 cup of the milk, and the vanilla. Set aside.
3. In a small bowl, mix together the flour, baking powder, salt, and cinnamon. Slowly combine the dry ingredients into the wet. Fold in the pecans.
4. Liberally spray a 7-inch springform pan with cooking spray. Pour the batter into the pan and place in the air fryer basket.
5. Bake for 30 to 35 minutes. While the cake is baking, in a small bowl, add the powdered sugar and whisk together with the remaining 6 teaspoons of milk. Set aside.
6. When the cake is done baking, remove the pan from the basket and let cool on a wire rack. After 10 minutes, remove and invert the cake from pan. Drizzle with the powdered sugar glaze and serve.

Roasted Vegetable Frittata

Servings: 1
Cooking Time: 19 Minutes

Ingredients:
- ½ red or green bell pepper, cut into ½-inch chunks
- 4 button mushrooms, sliced
- ½ cup diced zucchini
- ½ teaspoon chopped fresh oregano or thyme
- 1 teaspoon olive oil
- 3 eggs, beaten
- ½ cup grated Cheddar cheese
- salt and freshly ground black pepper, to taste
- 1 teaspoon butter
- 1 teaspoon chopped fresh parsley

Directions:
1. Preheat the air fryer to 400°F.
2. Toss the peppers, mushrooms, zucchini and oregano with the olive oil and air-fry for 6 minutes, shaking the basket once or twice during the cooking process to redistribute the ingredients.
3. While the vegetables are cooking, beat the eggs well in a bowl, stir in the Cheddar cheese and season with salt and freshly ground black pepper. Add the air-fried vegetables to this bowl when they have finished cooking.
4. Place a 6- or 7-inch non-stick metal cake pan into the air fryer basket with the butter using an aluminum sling to lower the pan into the basket. (Fold a piece of aluminum foil into a strip about 2-inches wide by 24-inches long.) Air-fry for 1 minute at 380°F to melt the butter. Remove the cake pan and rotate the pan to distribute the butter and grease the pan. Pour the egg mixture into the cake pan and return the pan to the air fryer, using the aluminum sling.
5. Air-fry at 380°F for 12 minutes, or until the frittata has puffed up and is lightly browned. Let the frittata sit in the air fryer for 5 minutes to cool to an edible temperature and set up. Remove the cake pan from the air fryer, sprinkle with parsley and serve immediately.

Fried Pb&j

Servings: 4
Cooking Time: 8 Minutes

Ingredients:
- ½ cup cornflakes, crushed
- ¼ cup shredded coconut
- 8 slices oat nut bread or any whole-grain, oversize bread
- 6 tablespoons peanut butter
- 2 medium bananas, cut into ½-inch-thick slices
- 6 tablespoons pineapple preserves
- 1 egg, beaten
- oil for misting or cooking spray

Directions:
1. Preheat air fryer to 360°F.
2. In a shallow dish, mix together the cornflake crumbs and coconut.
3. For each sandwich, spread one bread slice with 1½ tablespoons of peanut butter. Top with banana slices. Spread another bread slice with 1½ tablespoons of preserves. Combine to make a sandwich.
4. Using a pastry brush, brush top of sandwich lightly with beaten egg. Sprinkle with about 1½ tablespoons of crumb coating, pressing it in to make it stick. Spray with oil.
5. Turn sandwich over and repeat to coat and spray the other side.
6. Cooking 2 at a time, place sandwiches in air fryer basket and cook for 6 to 7minutes or until coating is golden brown and crispy. If sandwich doesn't brown enough, spray with a little more oil and cook at 390°F for another minute.
7. Cut cooked sandwiches in half and serve warm.

Buttermilk Biscuits

Servings: 4
Cooking Time: 9 Minutes

Ingredients:
- 1 cup flour
- 1½ teaspoons baking powder
- ¼ teaspoon baking soda
- ¼ teaspoon salt
- ¼ cup butter, cut into tiny cubes
- ¼ cup buttermilk, plus 2 tablespoons
- cooking spray

Directions:
1. Preheat air fryer to 330°F.
2. Combine flour, baking powder, soda, and salt in a medium bowl. Stir together.
3. Add cubed butter and cut into flour using knives or a pastry blender.
4. Add buttermilk and stir into a stiff dough.
5. Divide dough into 4 portions and shape each into a large biscuit. If dough is too sticky to handle, stir in 1 or 2 more tablespoons of flour before shaping. Biscuits should be firm enough to hold their shape. Otherwise they will stick to the air fryer basket.
6. Spray air fryer basket with nonstick cooking spray.
7. Place biscuits in basket and cook at 330°F for 9 minutes.

Sweet And Spicy Pumpkin Scones

Servings: 8
Cooking Time: 8 Minutes

Ingredients:
- 2 cups all-purpose flour
- 3 tablespoons packed brown sugar
- ½ teaspoon baking powder
- ¼ teaspoon baking soda
- ½ teaspoon kosher salt
- ½ teaspoon ground cinnamon
- ¼ teaspoon ground ginger
- ¼ teaspoon ground cardamom
- 4 tablespoons cold unsalted butter
- ½ cup plus 2 tablespoons pumpkin puree, divided
- 4 tablespoons milk, divided
- 1 large egg
- 1 cup powdered sugar

Directions:
1. In a large bowl, mix together the flour, brown sugar, baking powder, baking soda, salt, cinnamon, ginger, and cardamom. Using a pastry blender or two knives, cut in the butter until coarse crumbles appear.
2. In a small bowl, whisk together ½ cup of the pumpkin puree, 2 tablespoons of the milk, and the egg until combined. Pour the wet ingredients into the dry ingredients; stir to combine.
3. Form the dough into a ball and place onto a floured service. Press the dough out or use a rolling pin to roll out the dough until ½ inch thick and in a circle. Cut the dough into 8 wedges.
4. Bake at 360°F for 8 to 10 minutes or until completely cooked through. Cook in batches as needed.
5. In a medium bowl, whisk together the powdered sugar, the remaining 2 tablespoons of pumpkin puree, and the remaining 2 tablespoons of milk. When the pumpkin scones have cooled, drizzle the pumpkin glaze over the top before serving.

Appetizers And Snacks Recipes

Wrapped Shrimp Bites 18
Hot Cauliflower Bites 18
Brie-currant & Bacon Spread 18
Crunchy Pickle Chips 18
Buffalo Wings 19
Country Wings 19
Fried Dill Pickle Chips 19
Cheesy Spinach Dip 20
Sweet Plantain Chips 20
Avocado Toast With Lemony Shrimp 20
Jalapeño Poppers 21
Cheese Straws 21
Homemade Pretzel Bites 22
Shrimp Egg Rolls 22
Crispy Spiced Chickpeas 23
Chinese-style Potstickers 23
Crab Rangoon 23
Spanish Fried Baby Squid 24
Cheeseburger Slider Pockets 24
Orange-glazed Carrots 25
Spiced Parsnip Chips 25
Veggie Chips 25
Parmesan Crackers 26
Bbq Chips 26
Paprika Onion Blossom 26
Corn Dog Bites 27
Bacon Candy 27

Wrapped Shrimp Bites

Servings: 4
Cooking Time: 15 Minutes

Ingredients:
- 2 jumbo shrimp, peeled
- 2 bacon strips, sliced
- 2 tbsp lemon juice
- ½ tsp chipotle powder
- ½ tsp garlic salt

Directions:
1. Preheat air fryer to 350°F. Wrap the bacon around the shrimp and place the shrimp in the foil-lined frying basket, seam side down. Drizzle with lemon juice, chipotle powder and garlic salt. Air Fry for 10 minutes, turning the shrimp once until cooked through and bacon is crispy. Serve hot.

Hot Cauliflower Bites

Servings: 4
Cooking Time: 35 Minutes

Ingredients:
- 1 head cauliflower, cut into florets
- 1 cup all-purpose flour
- 1 tsp garlic powder
- 1/3 cup cayenne sauce

Directions:
1. Preheat air fryer to 370°F. Mix the flour, 1 cup of water, and garlic powder in a large bowl until a batter forms. Coat cauliflower in the batter, then transfer to a large bowl to drain excess. Place the cauliflower in the greased frying basket without stacking. Spray with cooking, then Bake for 6 minutes. Remove from the air fryer and transfer to a large bowl. Top with cayenne sauce. Return to the fryer and cook for 6 minutes or until crispy. Serve.

Brie-currant & Bacon Spread

Servings: 6
Cooking Time: 30 Minutes

Ingredients:
- 4 oz cream cheese, softened
- 3 tbsp mayonnaise
- 1 cup diced Brie cheese
- ½ tsp dried thyme
- 4 oz cooked bacon, crumbled
- 1/3 cup dried currants

Directions:
1. Preheat the air fryer to 350°F. Beat the cream cheese with the mayo until well blended. Stir in the Brie, thyme, bacon, and currants and pour the dip mix in a 6-inch round pan. Put the pan in the fryer and Air Fry for 10-12 minutes, stirring once until the dip is melting and bubbling. Serve warm.

Crunchy Pickle Chips

Servings: 4
Cooking Time: 20 Minutes

Ingredients:
- 1 lb dill pickles, sliced
- 2 eggs
- 1/3 cup flour
- 1/3 cup bread crumbs
- 1 tsp Italian seasoning

Directions:
1. Preheat air fryer to 400°F. Set out three small bowls. In the first bowl, add flour. In the second bowl, beat eggs. In the third bowl, mix bread crumbs with Italian seasoning. Dip the pickle slices in the flour. Shake, then dredge in egg. Roll in bread crumbs and shake excess. Place the pickles in the greased frying basket and Air Fry for 6 minutes. Flip them halfway through cooking and fry for another 3 minutes until crispy. Serve warm.

Buffalo Wings

Servings: 2
Cooking Time: 12 Minutes Per Batch

Ingredients:

- 2 pounds chicken wings
- 3 tablespoons butter, melted
- ¼ cup hot sauce (like Crystal® or Frank's®)
- Finishing Sauce:
- 3 tablespoons butter, melted
- ¼ cup hot sauce (like Crystal® or Frank's®)
- 1 teaspoon Worcestershire sauce

Directions:

1. Prepare the chicken wings by cutting off the wing tips and discarding (or freezing for chicken stock). Divide the drumettes from the wingettes by cutting through the joint. Place the chicken wing pieces in a large bowl.
2. Combine the melted butter and the hot sauce and stir to blend well. Pour the marinade over the chicken wings, cover and let the wings marinate for 2 hours or up to overnight in the refrigerator.
3. Preheat the air fryer to 400°F.
4. Air-fry the wings in two batches for 10 minutes per batch, shaking the basket halfway through the cooking process. When both batches are done, toss all the wings back into the basket for another 2 minutes to heat through and finish cooking.
5. While the wings are air-frying, combine the remaining 3 tablespoons of butter, ¼ cup of hot sauce and the Worcestershire sauce. Remove the wings from the air fryer, toss them in the finishing sauce and serve with some cooling blue cheese dip and celery sticks.

Country Wings

Servings: 4
Cooking Time: 19 Minutes

Ingredients:

- 2 pounds chicken wings
- Marinade
- 1 cup buttermilk
- ½ teaspoon black pepper
- ½ teaspoon salt
- Coating
- 1 cup flour

- 1 cup panko breadcrumbs
- 2 teaspoons salt
- 2 tablespoons poultry seasoning
- oil for misting or cooking spray

Directions:

1. Cut the tips off the wings. Discard or freeze for stock. Cut remaining wing sections apart at the joint to make 2 pieces per wing. Place wings in a large bowl or plastic bag.
2. Mix together all marinade ingredients and pour over wings. Refrigerate for at least 1 hour but for no more than 8 hours.
3. Preheat air fryer to 360°F.
4. Mix all coating ingredients together in a shallow dish or on wax paper.
5. Remove wings from marinade, shaking off excess, and roll in coating mixture.
6. Spray both sides of each wing with oil or cooking spray.
7. Place wings in air fryer basket in single layer, close but not too crowded. Cook for 19minutes or until chicken is done and juices run clear.
8. Repeat step 7 to cook remaining wings.

Fried Dill Pickle Chips

Servings: 4
Cooking Time: 12 Minutes

Ingredients:

- 1 cup All-purpose flour or tapioca flour
- 1 Large egg white(s)
- 1 tablespoon Brine from a jar of dill pickles
- 1 cup Seasoned Italian-style dried bread crumbs (gluten-free, if a concern)
- 2 Large dill pickle(s) (8 to 10 inches long), cut into ½-inch-thick rounds
- Vegetable oil spray

Directions:

1. Preheat the air fryer to 400°F.
2. Set up and fill three shallow soup plates or small pie plates on your counter: one for the flour, one for the egg white(s) whisked with the pickle brine, and one for the bread crumbs.
3. Set a pickle round in the flour and turn it to coat all sides, even the edge. Gently shake off the excess flour, then dip the round into the egg-white mixture and turn to coat both sides and the edge. Let any excess egg white mixture slip back into the rest, then set the round in the

bread crumbs and turn it to coat both sides as well as the edge. Set aside on a cutting board and soldier on, dipping and coating the remaining rounds. Lightly coat the coated rounds on both sides with vegetable oil spray.

4. Set the pickle rounds in the basket in one layer. Air-fry undisturbed for 7 minutes, or until golden brown and crunchy. Cool in the basket for a few minutes before using kitchen tongs to transfer the (still hot) rounds to a serving platter.

Cheesy Spinach Dip

Servings: 6
Cooking Time: 35 Minutes

Ingredients:
- ½ can refrigerated breadstick dough
- 8 oz feta cheese, cubed
- ¼ cup sour cream
- ½ cup baby spinach
- ½ cup grated Swiss cheese
- 2 green onions, chopped
- 2 tbsp melted butter
- 4 tsp grated Parmesan cheese

Directions:
1. Preheat air fryer to 320°F. Blend together feta, sour cream, spinach, Swiss cheese, and green onions in a bowl. Spread into the pan and Bake until hot, about 8 minutes. Unroll six of the breadsticks and cut in half crosswise to make 12 pieces. Carefully stretch each piece and tie into a loose knot. Tuck in the ends to prevent burning.
2. When the dip is ready, remove the pan from the air fryer and place each bread knot on top of the dip until the dip is covered. Brush melted butter on each knot and sprinkle with Parmesan. Bake until the knots are golden, 8-13 minutes. Serve warm.

Sweet Plantain Chips

Servings: 4
Cooking Time: 11 Minutes

Ingredients:
- 2 Very ripe plantain(s), peeled and sliced into 1-inch pieces
- Vegetable oil spray

- 3 tablespoons Maple syrup
- For garnishing Coarse sea salt or kosher salt

Directions:
1. Pour about ½ cup water into the bottom of your air fryer basket or into a metal tray on a lower rack in some models. Preheat the air fryer to 400°F.
2. Put the plantain pieces in a bowl, coat them with vegetable oil spray, and toss gently, spraying at least one more time and tossing repeatedly, until the pieces are well coated.
3. When the machine is at temperature, arrange the plantain pieces in the basket in one layer. Air-fry undisturbed for 5 minutes.
4. Remove the basket from the machine and spray the back of a metal spatula with vegetable oil spray. Use the spatula to press down on the plantain pieces, spraying it again as needed, to flatten the pieces to about half their original height. Brush the plantain pieces with maple syrup, then return the basket to the machine and continue air-frying undisturbed for 6 minutes, or until the plantain pieces are soft and caramelized.
5. Use kitchen tongs to transfer the pieces to a serving platter. Sprinkle the pieces with salt and cool for a couple of minutes before serving. Or cool to room temperature before serving, about 1 hour.

Avocado Toast With Lemony Shrimp

Servings: 4
Cooking Time: 6 Minutes

Ingredients:
- 6 ounces Raw medium shrimp (30 to 35 per pound), peeled and deveined
- 1½ teaspoons Finely grated lemon zest
- 2 teaspoons Lemon juice
- 1½ teaspoons Minced garlic
- 1½ teaspoons Ground black pepper
- 4 Rye or whole-wheat bread slices (gluten-free, if a concern)
- 2 Ripe Hass avocado(s), halved, pitted, peeled and roughly chopped
- For garnishing Coarse sea salt or kosher salt

Directions:
1. Preheat the air fryer to 400°F.
2. Toss the shrimp, lemon zest, lemon juice,

garlic, and pepper in a bowl until the shrimp are evenly coated.

3. When the machine is at temperature, use kitchen tongs to place the shrimp in a single layer in the basket. Air-fry undisturbed for 4 minutes, or until the shrimp are pink and barely firm. Use kitchen tongs to transfer the shrimp to a cutting board.

4. Working in batches, set as many slices of bread as will fit in the basket in one layer. Air-fry undisturbed for 2 minutes, just until warmed through and crisp. The bread will not brown much.

5. Arrange the bread slices on a clean, dry work surface. Divide the avocado bits among them and gently smash the avocado into a coarse paste with the tines of a flatware fork. Top the toasts with the shrimp and sprinkle with salt as a garnish.

veins. Stir a small amount into filling, taste, and continue adding a little at a time until filling is as hot as you like.

5. Stuff each pepper slice with filling.

6. Place cornstarch in a shallow dish.

7. In another shallow dish, beat together egg and lime juice.

8. Place breadcrumbs and salt in a third shallow dish and stir together.

9. Dip each pepper slice in cornstarch, shake off excess, then dip in egg mixture.

10. Roll in breadcrumbs, pressing to make coating stick.

11. Place pepper slices on a plate in single layer and freeze them for 30minutes.

12. Preheat air fryer to 390°F.

13. Spray frozen peppers with oil or cooking spray. Place in air fryer basket in a single layer and cook for 5minutes.

Jalapeño Poppers

Servings: 18
Cooking Time: 5 Minutes

Ingredients:
- ½ pound jalapeño peppers
- ¼ cup cornstarch
- 1 egg
- 1 tablespoon lime juice
- ¼ cup plain breadcrumbs
- ¼ cup panko breadcrumbs
- ½ teaspoon salt
- oil for misting or cooking spray
- Filling
- 4 ounces cream cheese
- 1 teaspoon grated lime zest
- ¼ teaspoon chile powder
- ⅛ teaspoon garlic powder
- ¼ teaspoon salt

Directions:
1. Combine all filling ingredients in small bowl and mix well. Refrigerate while preparing peppers.

2. Cut jalapeños into ½-inch lengthwise slices. Use a small, sharp knife to remove seeds and veins.

3. a. For mild appetizers, discard seeds and veins.

4. b. For hot appetizers, finely chop seeds and

Cheese Straws

Servings: 8
Cooking Time: 7 Minutes

Ingredients:
- For dusting All-purpose flour
- Two quarters of one thawed sheet (that is, a half of the sheet cut into two even pieces; wrap and refreeze the remainder) A 17.25-ounce box frozen puff pastry
- 1 Large egg(s)
- 2 tablespoons Water
- ¼ cup (about ¾ ounce) Finely grated Parmesan cheese
- up to 1 teaspoon Ground black pepper

Directions:
1. Preheat the air fryer to 400°F.

2. Dust a clean, dry work surface with flour. Set one of the pieces of puff pastry on top, dust the pastry lightly with flour, and roll with a rolling pin to a 6-inch square.

3. Whisk the egg(s) and water in a small or medium bowl until uniform. Brush the pastry square(s) generously with this mixture. Sprinkle each square with 2 tablespoons grated cheese and up to ½ teaspoon ground black pepper.

4. Cut each square into 4 even strips. Grasp each end of 1 strip with clean, dry hands; twist it into a cheese straw. Place the twisted straws

on a baking sheet.

5. Lay as many straws as will fit in the air-fryer basket—as a general rule, 4 of them in a small machine, 5 in a medium model, or 6 in a large. There should be space for air to circulate around the straws. Set the baking sheet with any remaining straws in the fridge.

6. Air-fry undisturbed for 7 minutes, or until puffed and crisp. Use tongs to transfer the cheese straws to a wire rack, then make subsequent batches in the same way (keeping the baking sheet with the remaining straws in the fridge as each batch cooks). Serve warm.

Homemade Pretzel Bites

Servings: 8
Cooking Time: 6 Minutes

Ingredients:
- 4¾ cups filtered water, divided
- 1 tablespoon butter
- 1 package fast-rising yeast
- ½ teaspoon salt
- 2⅓ cups bread flour
- 2 tablespoons baking soda
- 2 egg whites
- 1 teaspoon kosher salt

Directions:
1. Preheat the air fryer to 370°F.
2. In a large microwave-safe bowl, add ¾ cup of the water. Heat for 40 seconds in the microwave. Remove and whisk in the butter; then mix in the yeast and salt. Let sit 5 minutes.
3. Using a stand mixer with a dough hook attachment, add the yeast liquid and mix in the bread flour ⅓ cup at a time until all the flour is added and a dough is formed.
4. Remove the bowl from the stand; then let the dough rise 1 hour in a warm space, covered with a kitchen towel.
5. After the dough has doubled in size, remove from the bowl and punch down a few times on a lightly floured flat surface.
6. Divide the dough into 4 balls; then roll each ball out into a long, skinny, sticklike shape. Using a sharp knife, cut each dough stick into 6 pieces.
7. Repeat Step 6 for the remaining dough balls until you have about 24 bites formed.

8. Heat the remaining 4 cups of water over the stovetop in a medium pot with the baking soda stirred in.
9. Drop the pretzel bite dough into the hot water and let boil for 60 seconds, remove, and let slightly cool.
10. Lightly brush the top of each bite with the egg whites, and then cover with a pinch of kosher salt.
11. Spray the air fryer basket with olive oil spray and place the pretzel bites on top. Cook for 6 to 8 minutes, or until lightly browned. Remove and keep warm.
12. Repeat until all pretzel bites are cooked.
13. Serve warm.

Shrimp Egg Rolls

Servings: 8
Cooking Time: 10 Minutes

Ingredients:
- 1 tablespoon vegetable oil
- ½ head green or savoy cabbage, finely shredded
- 1 cup shredded carrots
- 1 cup canned bean sprouts, drained
- 1 tablespoon soy sauce
- ½ teaspoon sugar
- 1 teaspoon sesame oil
- ¼ cup hoisin sauce
- freshly ground black pepper
- 1 pound cooked shrimp, diced
- ¼ cup scallions
- 8 egg roll wrappers
- vegetable oil
- duck sauce

Directions:
1. Preheat a large sauté pan over medium-high heat. Add the oil and cook the cabbage, carrots and bean sprouts until they start to wilt – about 3 minutes. Add the soy sauce, sugar, sesame oil, hoisin sauce and black pepper. Sauté for a few more minutes. Stir in the shrimp and scallions and cook until the vegetables are just tender. Transfer the mixture to a colander in a bowl to cool. Press or squeeze out any excess water from the filling so that you don't end up with soggy egg rolls.
2. To make the egg rolls, place the egg roll

wrappers on a flat surface with one of the points facing towards you so they look like diamonds. Dividing the filling evenly between the eight wrappers, spoon the mixture onto the center of the egg roll wrappers. Spread the filling across the center of the wrappers from the left corner to the right corner, but leave 2 inches from each corner empty. Brush the empty sides of the wrapper with a little water. Fold the bottom corner of the wrapper tightly up over the filling, trying to avoid making any air pockets. Fold the left corner in toward the center and then the right corner toward the center. It should now look like an envelope. Tightly roll the egg roll from the bottom to the top open corner. Press to seal the egg roll together, brushing with a little extra water if need be. Repeat this technique with all 8 egg rolls.

3. Preheat the air fryer to 370°F.
4. Spray or brush all sides of the egg rolls with vegetable oil. Air-fry four egg rolls at a time for 10 minutes, turning them over halfway through the cooking time.
5. Serve hot with duck sauce or your favorite dipping sauce.

Crispy Spiced Chickpeas

Servings: 2
Cooking Time: 20 Minutes

Ingredients:
• 1 (15-ounce) can chickpeas, drained (or 1½ cups cooked chickpeas)
• ½ teaspoon salt
• ½ teaspoon chili powder
• ¼ teaspoon ground cinnamon
• ⅛ teaspoon smoked paprika
• pinch ground cayenne pepper
• 1 tablespoon olive oil

Directions:
1. Preheat the air fryer to 400°F.
2. Dry the chickpeas as well as you can with a clean kitchen towel, rubbing off any loose skins as necessary. Combine the spices in a small bowl. Toss the chickpeas with the olive oil and then add the spices and toss again.
3. Air-fry for 15 minutes, shaking the basket a couple of times while they cook.
4. Check the chickpeas to see if they are crispy

enough and if necessary, air-fry for another 5 minutes to crisp them further. Serve warm, or cool to room temperature and store in an airtight container for up to two weeks.

Chinese-style Potstickers

Servings: 6
Cooking Time: 30 Minutes

Ingredients:
• 1 cup shredded Chinese cabbage
• ¼ cup chopped shiitake mushrooms
• ¼ cup grated carrots
• 2 tbsp minced chives
• 2 garlic cloves, minced
• 2 tsp grated fresh ginger
• 12 dumpling wrappers
• 2 tsp sesame oil

Directions:
1. Preheat air fryer to 370°F. Toss the Chinese cabbage, shiitake mushrooms, carrots, chives, garlic, and ginger in a baking pan and stir. Place the pan in the fryer and Bake for 3-6 minutes. Put a dumpling wrapper on a clean workspace, then top with a tablespoon of the veggie mix.
2. Fold the wrapper in half to form a half-circle and use water to seal the edges. Repeat with remaining wrappers and filling. Brush the potstickers with sesame oil and arrange them on the frying basket. Air Fry for 5 minutes until the bottoms should are golden brown. Take the pan out, add 1 tbsp of water, and put it back in the fryer to Air Fry for 4-6 minutes longer. Serve hot.

Crab Rangoon

Servings: 18
Cooking Time: 6 Minutes

Ingredients:
• 4½ tablespoons (a little more than ¼ pound) Crabmeat, preferably backfin or claw, picked over for shells and cartilage
• 1½ ounces (3 tablespoons) Regular or low-fat cream cheese (not fat-free), softened to room temperature
• 1½ tablespoons Minced scallion
• 1½ teaspoons Minced garlic
• 1½ teaspoons Worcestershire sauce
• 18 Wonton wrappers (thawed, if necessary)

- Vegetable oil spray

Directions:

1. Preheat the air fryer to 400°F.
2. Gently stir the crab, cream cheese, scallion, garlic, and Worcestershire sauce in a medium bowl until well combined.
3. Set a bowl of water on a clean, dry work surface or next to a large cutting board. Set one wonton wrapper on the surface, then put a teaspoonful of the crab mixture in the center of the wrapper. Dip your clean finger in the water and run it around the edge of the wrapper. Bring all four sides up to the center and over the filling, and pinch them together in the middle to seal without covering all of the filling. The traditional look is for the corners of the filled wonton to become four open "flower petals" radiating out from the filled center. Set the filled wonton aside and continue making more as needed. (If you want a video tutorial on filling these, see ours at our YouTube channel, Cooking with Bruce and Mark.)
4. Generously coat the filled wontons with vegetable oil spray. Set them sealed side up in the basket with a little room among them. Air-fry undisturbed for 6 minutes, or until golden brown and crisp.
5. Use a nonstick-safe spatula to gently transfer the wontons to a wire rack. Cool for 5 minutes before serving warm.

Spanish Fried Baby Squid

Servings: 2
Cooking Time: 30 Minutes

Ingredients:

- 1 cup baby squid
- ½ cup semolina flour
- ½ tsp Spanish paprika
- ½ tsp garlic powder
- 2 eggs
- Salt and pepper to taste
- 2 tbsp lemon juice
- 1 tsp Old Bay seasoning

Directions:

1. Preheat air fryer to 350°F. Beat the eggs in a bowl. Stir in lemon juice and set aside. Mix flour, Old Bay seasoning, garlic powder, paprika, salt, and pepper in another bowl. Dip each piece of squid into the flour, then into the eggs, and then again. Transfer them to the greased frying basket and Air Fry for 18-20 minutes, shaking the basket occasionally until crispy and golden brown. Serve hot.

Cheeseburger Slider Pockets

Servings: 4
Cooking Time: 13 Minutes

Ingredients:

- 1 pound extra lean ground beef
- 2 teaspoons steak seasoning
- 2 tablespoons Worcestershire sauce
- 8 ounces Cheddar cheese
- ⅓ cup ketchup
- ¼ cup light mayonnaise
- 1 tablespoon pickle relish
- 1 pound frozen bread dough, defrosted
- 1 egg, beaten
- sesame seeds
- vegetable or olive oil, in a spray bottle

Directions:

1. Combine the ground beef, steak seasoning and Worcestershire sauce in a large bowl. Divide the meat mixture into 12 equal portions. Cut the Cheddar cheese into twelve 2-inch squares, about ¼-inch thick. Stuff a square of cheese into the center of each portion of meat and shape into a 3-inch patty.
2. Make the slider sauce by combining the ketchup, mayonnaise, and relish in a small bowl. Set aside.
3. Cut the bread dough into twelve pieces. Shape each piece of dough into a ball and use a rolling pin to roll them out into 4-inch circles. Dollop ½ teaspoon of the slider sauce into the center of each dough circle. Place a beef patty on top of the sauce and wrap the dough around the patty, pinching the dough together to seal the pocket shut. Try not to stretch the dough too much when bringing the edges together. Brush both sides of the slider pocket with the beaten egg. Sprinkle sesame seeds on top of each pocket.
4. Preheat the air fryer to 350°F.
5. Spray or brush the bottom of the air fryer basket with oil. Air-fry the slider pockets four at a time. Transfer the slider pockets to the

air fryer basket, seam side down and air-fry at 350°F for 10 minutes, until the dough is golden brown. Flip the slider pockets over and air-fry for another 3 minutes. When all the batches are done, pop all the sliders into the air fryer for a few minutes to re-heat and serve them hot out of the fryer.

Orange-glazed Carrots

Servings: 3
Cooking Time: 25 Minutes

Ingredients:

- 3 carrots, cut into spears
- 1 tbsp orange juice
- 2 tsp balsamic vinegar
- 1 tsp avocado oil
- 1 tsp clear honey
- ½ tsp dried rosemary
- ¼ tsp salt
- ¼ tsp lemon zest

Directions:

1. Preheat air fryer to 390°F. Put the carrots in a baking pan. Add the orange juice, balsamic vinegar, oil, honey, rosemary, salt, and zest. Stir well. Roast for 15-18 minutes, shaking them once or twice until the carrots are bright orange, glazed, and tender. Serve while hot.

Spiced Parsnip Chips

Servings:2
Cooking Time: 35 Minutes

Ingredients:

- ½ tsp smoked paprika
- ¼ tsp chili powder
- ¼ tsp garlic powder
- ⅛ tsp onion powder
- ⅛ tsp cayenne pepper
- ⅛ tsp granulated sugar
- 1 tsp salt
- 1 parsnip, cut into chips
- 2 tsp olive oil

Directions:

1. Preheat air fryer to 400ºF. Mix all spices in a bowl and reserve. In another bowl, combine parsnip chips, olive oil, and salt. Place parsnip chips in the lightly greased frying basket and Air Fry for 12 minutes, shaking once. Transfer the chips to a bowl, toss in seasoning mix, and let sit for 15 minutes before serving.

Veggie Chips

Servings: X
Cooking Time: X

Ingredients:

- sweet potato
- large parsnip
- large carrot
- turnip
- large beet
- vegetable or canola oil, in a spray bottle
- salt

Directions:

1. You can do a medley of vegetable chips, or just select from the vegetables listed. Whatever you choose to do, scrub the vegetables well and then slice them paper-thin using a mandolin (about -1/16 inch thick).
2. Preheat the air fryer to 400°F.
3. Air-fry the chips in batches, one type of vegetable at a time. Spray the chips lightly with oil and transfer them to the air fryer basket. The key is to NOT over-load the basket. You can overlap the chips a little, but don't pile them on top of each other. Doing so will make it much harder to get evenly browned and crispy chips. Air-fry at 400°F for the time indicated below, shaking the basket several times during the cooking process for even cooking.
4. Sweet Potato – 8 to 9 minutes
5. Parsnips – 5 minutes
6. Carrot – 7 minutes
7. Turnips – 8 minutes
8. Beets – 9 minutes
9. Season the chips with salt during the last couple of minutes of air-frying. Check the chips as they cook until they are done to your liking. Some will start to brown sooner than others.
10. You can enjoy the chips warm out of the air fryer or cool them to room temperature for crispier chips.

Parmesan Crackers

Servings: 6
Cooking Time: 6 Minutes

Ingredients:
- 2 cups finely grated Parmesan cheese
- ¼ teaspoon paprika
- ¼ teaspoon garlic powder
- ½ teaspoon dried thyme
- 1 tablespoon all-purpose flour

Directions:
1. Preheat the air fryer to 380°F.
2. In a medium bowl, stir together the Parmesan, paprika, garlic powder, thyme, and flour.
3. Line the air fryer basket with parchment paper.
4. Using a tablespoon measuring tool, create 1-tablespoon mounds of seasoned cheese on the parchment paper, leaving 2 inches between the mounds to allow for spreading.
5. Cook the crackers for 6 minutes. Allow the cheese to harden and cool before handling. Repeat in batches with the remaining cheese.

Bbq Chips

Servings: 2
Cooking Time: 30 Minutes

Ingredients:
- 1 scrubbed russet potato, sliced
- ½ tsp smoked paprika
- ¼ tsp chili powder
- ¼ tsp garlic powder
- 1/8 tsp onion powder
- ¼ tbsp smoked paprika
- 1/8 tsp light brown sugar
- Salt and pepper to taste
- 2 tsp olive oil

Directions:
1. Preheat air fryer at 400°F. Combine all seasoning in a bowl. Set aside. In another bowl, mix potato chips, olive oil, black pepper, and salt until coated. Place potato chips in the frying basket and Air Fry for 17 minutes, shaking 3 times. Transfer it into a bowl. Sprinkle with the bbq mixture and let sit for 15 minutes. Serve immediately.

Paprika Onion Blossom

Servings: 4
Cooking Time: 35 Minutes + Cooling Time

Ingredients:
- 1 large onion
- 1 ½ cups flour
- 1 tsp garlic powder
- 1 tsp paprika
- ½ tsp bell pepper powder
- Salt and pepper to taste
- 2 eggs
- 1 cup milk

Directions:
1. Remove the tip of the onion but leave the root base intact. Peel the onion to the root and remove skin. Place the onion cut-side down on a cutting board. Starting ½-inch down from the root, cut down to the bottom. Repeat until the onion is divided into quarters. Starting ½-inch down from the root, repeat the cuts in between the first cuts. Repeat this process in between the cuts until you have 16 cuts in the onion. Flip the onion onto the root and carefully spread the inner layers. Set aside.
2. In a bowl, add flour, garlic, paprika, bell pepper, salt, and pepper, then stir. In another large bowl, whisk eggs and milk. Place the onion in the flour bowl and cover with flour mixture. Transfer the onion into the egg mixture and coat completely with either a spoon or basting brush. Return the onion to the flour bowl and cover completely. Take a sheet of foil and wrap the onion with the foil. Freeze for 45 minutes.
3. Preheat air fryer to 400°F. Remove the onion from the foil and place in the greased frying basket. Air Fry for 10 minutes. Lightly spray the onion with cooking oil, then cook for another 10-15 minutes. Serve immediately.

Corn Dog Bites

Servings: 3
Cooking Time: 12 Minutes

Ingredients:
- 3 cups Purchased cornbread stuffing mix
- ⅓ cup All-purpose flour
- 2 Large egg(s), well beaten
- 3 Hot dogs, cut into 2-inch pieces (vegetarian hot dogs, if preferred)
- Vegetable oil spray

Directions:
1. Preheat the air fryer to 375°F.
2. Put the cornbread stuffing mix in a food processor. Cover and pulse to grind into a mixture like fine bread crumbs.
3. Set up and fill three shallow soup plates or small pie plates on your counter: one for the flour, one for the egg(s), and one for the stuffing mix crumbs.
4. Dip a hot dog piece in the flour to coat it completely, then gently shake off any excess. Dip the hot dog piece into the egg(s) and gently roll it around to coat all surfaces, then pick it up and allow any excess egg to slip back into the rest. Set the hot dog piece in the stuffing mix crumbs and roll it gently to coat it evenly and well on all sides, even the ends. Set it aside on a cutting board and continue dipping and coating the remaining hot dog pieces.
5. Give the coated hot dog pieces a generous coating of vegetable oil spray on all sides, then set them in the basket in one layer with some space between them. Air-fry undisturbed for 10 minutes, or until golden brown and crunchy. (You'll need to add 2 minutes in the air fryer if the temperature is at 360°F.)
6. Use a nonstick-safe spatula, and perhaps a flatware fork for balance, to transfer the corn dog bites to a wire rack. Cool for 5 minutes before serving.

Bacon Candy

Servings: 6
Cooking Time: 6 Minutes

Ingredients:
- 1½ tablespoons Honey
- 1 teaspoon White wine vinegar
- 3 Extra thick-cut bacon strips, halved widthwise (gluten-free, if a concern)
- ½ teaspoon Ground black pepper

Directions:
1. Preheat the air fryer to 350°F.
2. Whisk the honey and vinegar in a small bowl until incorporated.
3. When the machine is at temperature, remove the basket. Lay the bacon strip halves in the basket in one layer. Brush the tops with the honey mixture; sprinkle each bacon strip evenly with black pepper.
4. Return the basket to the machine and air-fry undisturbed for 6 minutes, or until the bacon is crunchy. Or a little less time if you prefer bacon that's still pliable, an extra minute if you want the bacon super crunchy. Take care that the honey coating doesn't burn. Remove the basket from the machine and set aside for 5 minutes. Use kitchen tongs to transfer the bacon strips to a serving plate.

Beef ,pork & Lamb Recipes

Cinnamon-stick Kofta Skewers 29
Hungarian Pork Burgers 29
Wiener Schnitzel 29
Skirt Steak With Horseradish Cream 30
Cowboy Rib Eye Steak 30
Steakhouse Burgers With Red Onion Compote 30
Beef Short Ribs..31
Lemon Pork Escalopes 31
Delicious Juicy Pork Meatballs 31
Authentic Sausage Kartoffel Salad 32
Spicy Hoisin Bbq Pork Chops 32
Zesty London Broil 32
Peppered Steak Bites 33
Sriracha Short Ribs 33
Stuffed Pork Chops..33
Sirloin Steak Flatbread...34
Chinese-style Lamb Chops...34
Peachy Pork Chops 34
Korean-style Lamb Shoulder Chops 35
Friday Night Cheeseburgers 35
Taco Pie With Meatballs..35
Balsamic Marinated Rib Eye Steak With Balsamic Fried
Cipollini Onions 36
Ground Beef Calzones..36
Sweet And Sour Pork..36
Pork Chops 37
Better-than-chinese-take-out Sesame Beef...................37
Asian-style Flank Steak 38

BEEF, PORK & LAMB RECIPES

Cinnamon-stick Kofta Skewers

Servings: 8
Cooking Time: 15 Minutes

Ingredients:
- 1 pound Lean ground beef
- ½ teaspoon Ground cumin
- ½ teaspoon Onion powder
- ½ teaspoon Ground dried turmeric
- ½ teaspoon Ground cinnamon
- ½ teaspoon Table salt
- Up to a ⅛ teaspoon Cayenne
- 8 3½- to 4-inch-long cinnamon sticks (see the headnote)
- Vegetable oil spray

Directions:
1. Preheat the air fryer to 375°F .
2. Gently mix the ground beef, cumin, onion powder, turmeric, cinnamon, salt, and cayenne in a bowl until the meat is evenly mixed with the spices. (Clean, dry hands work best!) Divide this mixture into 2-ounce portions, each about the size of a golf ball.
3. Wrap one portion of the meat mixture around a cinnamon stick, using about three-quarters of the length of the stick, covering one end but leaving a little "handle" of cinnamon stick protruding from the other end. Set aside and continue making more kofta skewers.
4. Generously coat the formed kofta skewers on all sides with vegetable oil spray. Set them in the basket with as much air space between them as possible. Air-fry undisturbed for 13 minutes, or until browned and cooked through. If the machine is at 360°F, you may need to add 2 minutes to the cooking time.
5. Use a nonstick-safe spatula, and perhaps kitchen tongs for balance, to gently transfer the kofta skewers to a wire rack. Cool for at least 5 minutes or up to 20 minutes before serving.

Hungarian Pork Burgers

Servings: 4
Cooking Time: 30 Minutes

Ingredients:
- 8 sandwich buns, halved
- ½ cup mayonnaise
- 2 tbsp mustard
- 1 tbsp lemon juice
- ¼ cup sliced red cabbage
- ¼ cup grated carrots
- 1 lb ground pork
- ½ tsp Hungarian paprika
- 1 cup lettuce, torn
- 2 tomatoes, sliced

Directions:
1. Mix the mayonnaise, 1 tbsp of mustard, lemon juice, cabbage, and carrots in a bowl. Refrigerate for 10 minutes.
2. Preheat air fryer to 400°F. Toss the pork, remaining mustard, and paprika in a bowl, mix, then make 8 patties. Place them in the air fryer and Air Fry for 7-9 minutes, flipping once until cooked through. Put some lettuce on one bottom bun, then top with a tomato slice, one burger, and some cabbage mix. Put another bun on top and serve. Repeat for all burgers. Serve and enjoy!

Wiener Schnitzel

Servings: 4
Cooking Time: 14 Minutes

Ingredients:
- 4 thin boneless pork loin chops
- 2 tablespoons lemon juice
- ½ cup flour
- 1 teaspoon salt
- ¼ teaspoon marjoram
- 1 cup plain breadcrumbs
- 2 eggs, beaten
- oil for misting or cooking spray

Directions:

1. Rub the lemon juice into all sides of pork chops.
2. Mix together the flour, salt, and marjoram.
3. Place flour mixture on a sheet of wax paper.
4. Place breadcrumbs on another sheet of wax paper.
5. Roll pork chops in flour, dip in beaten eggs, then roll in breadcrumbs. Mist all sides with oil or cooking spray.
6. Spray air fryer basket with nonstick cooking spray and place pork chops in basket.
7. Cook at 390°F for 7minutes. Turn, mist again, and cook for another 7 minutes, until well done. Serve with lemon wedges.

Skirt Steak With Horseradish Cream

Servings:2
Cooking Time: 20 Minutes

Ingredients:
- 1 cup heavy cream
- 3 tbsp horseradish sauce
- 1 lemon, zested
- 1 skirt steak, halved
- 2 tbsp olive oil
- Salt and pepper to taste

Directions:
1. Mix together the heavy cream, horseradish sauce, and lemon zest in a small bowl. Let chill in the fridge.
2. Preheat air fryer to 400ºF. Brush steak halves with olive oil and sprinkle with salt and pepper. Place steaks in the frying basket and Air Fry for 10 minutes or until you reach your desired doneness, flipping once. Let sit onto a cutting board for 5 minutes.Thinly slice against the grain and divide between 2 plates. Drizzle with the horseradish sauce over. Serve and enjoy!

Cowboy Rib Eye Steak

Servings:2
Cooking Time: 20 Minutes

Ingredients:
- ¼ cup barbecue sauce
- 1 clove garlic, minced
- ⅛ tsp chili pepper
- ¼ tsp sweet paprika
- ¼ tsp cumin
- 1 rib-eye steak

Directions:
1. Preheat air fryer to 400ºF. In a bowl, whisk the barbecue sauce, garlic, chili pepper, paprika, and cumin. Divide in half and brush the steak with half of the sauce. Add steak to the lightly greased frying basket and Air Fry for 10 minutes until you reach your desired doneness, turning once and brushing with the remaining sauce. Let rest for 5 minutes onto a cutting board before slicing. Serve warm.

Steakhouse Burgers With Red Onion Compote

Servings: 4
Cooking Time: 22 Minutes

Ingredients:
- 1½ pounds lean ground beef
- 2 cloves garlic, minced and divided
- 1 teaspoon Worcestershire sauce
- 1 teaspoon sea salt, divided
- ½ teaspoon black pepper
- 1 tablespoon extra-virgin olive oil
- 1 red onion, thinly sliced
- ¼ cup balsamic vinegar
- 1 teaspoon sugar
- 1 tablespoon tomato paste
- 2 tablespoons mayonnaise
- 2 tablespoons sour cream
- 4 brioche hamburger buns
- 1 cup arugula

Directions:
1. In a large bowl, mix together the ground beef, 1 of the minced garlic cloves, the Worcestershire sauce, ½ teaspoon of the salt, and the black pepper. Form the meat into 1-inch-thick patties. Make a dent in the center (this helps the center cook evenly). Let the meat sit for 15 minutes.
2. Meanwhile, in a small saucepan over medium heat, cook the olive oil and red onion for 4 minutes, stirring frequently to avoid burning. Add in the balsamic vinegar, sugar, and tomato paste, and cook for an additional 3 minutes, stirring frequently. Transfer the onion compote to a small bowl.
3. Preheat the air fryer to 350°F.
4. In another small bowl, mix together the re-

maining minced garlic, the mayonnaise, and the sour cream. Spread the mayo mixture on the insides of the brioche buns.

5. Cook the hamburgers for 6 minutes, flip the burgers, and cook an additional 2 to 6 minutes. Check the internal temperature to avoid under- or overcooking. Hamburgers should be cooked to at least 160°F. After cooking, cover with foil and let the meat rest for 5 minutes.

6. Meanwhile, place the buns inside the air fryer and toast them for 3 minutes.

7. To assemble the burgers, place the hamburger on one side of the bun, top with onion compote and ¼ cup arugula, and then place the other half of the bun on top.

Beef Short Ribs

Servings: 4
Cooking Time: 20 Minutes

Ingredients:
- 2 tablespoons soy sauce
- 1 tablespoon sesame oil
- 2 tablespoons brown sugar
- 1 teaspoon ground ginger
- 2 garlic cloves, crushed
- 1 pound beef short ribs

Directions:
1. In a small bowl, mix together the soy sauce, sesame oil, brown sugar, and ginger. Transfer the mixture to a large resealable plastic bag, and place the garlic cloves and short ribs into the bag. Secure and place in the refrigerator for an hour (or overnight).

2. When you're ready to prepare the dish, preheat the air fryer to 330°F.

3. Liberally spray the air fryer basket with olive oil mist and set the beef short ribs in the basket.

4. Cook for 10 minutes, flip the short ribs, and then cook another 10 minutes.

5. Remove the short ribs from the air fryer basket, loosely cover with aluminum foil, and let them rest. The short ribs will continue to cook after they're removed from the basket. Check the internal temperature after 5 minutes to make sure it reached 145°F if you prefer a well-done meat. If it didn't reach 145°F and you would like it to be cooked longer, you can put it back into the air fryer basket at 330°F for an-

other 3 minutes.

6. Remove from the basket and let it rest, covered with aluminum foil, for 5 minutes. Serve immediately.

Lemon Pork Escalopes

Servings: 4
Cooking Time: 45 Minutes

Ingredients:
- 4 pork loin chops
- 1 cup breadcrumbs
- 2 eggs, beaten
- Salt and pepper to taste
- ½ tbsp thyme, chopped
- ½ tsp smoked paprika
- ½ tsp ground cumin
- 1 lemon, zested

Directions:
1. Preheat air fryer to 350°F. Mix the breadcrumbs, thyme, smoked paprika, cumin, lemon zest, salt, and pepper in a bowl. Add the pork chops and toss to coat. Dip in the beaten eggs, then dip again into the dry ingredients. Place the coated chops in the greased frying basket and Air Fry for 16-18 minutes, turning once. Serve and enjoy!

Delicious Juicy Pork Meatballs

Servings: 4
Cooking Time: 35 Minutes

Ingredients:
- ¼ cup grated cheddar cheese
- 1 lb ground pork
- 1 egg
- 1 tbsp Greek yogurt
- ½ tsp onion powder
- ¼ cup chopped parsley
- 2 tbsp bread crumbs
- ¼ tsp garlic powder
- Salt and pepper to taste

Directions:
1. Preheat air fryer to 350°F. In a bowl, combine the ground pork, egg, yogurt, onion, parsley, cheddar cheese, bread crumbs, garlic, salt, and black pepper. Form mixture into 16 meatballs. Place meatballs in the lightly greased frying basket and Air Fry for 8-10 minutes, flipping once.

Serve.

Authentic Sausage Kartoffel Salad

Servings: 4
Cooking Time: 50 Minutes

Ingredients:
- ½ lb cooked Polish sausage, sliced
- 2 cooked potatoes, cubed
- 1 cup chicken broth
- 2 tbsp olive oil
- 1 onion, chopped
- 2 garlic cloves, minced
- ¼ cup apple cider vinegar
- 3 tbsp light brown sugar
- 2 tbsp cornstarch
- ¼ cup sour cream
- 1 tsp yellow mustard
- 2 tbsp chopped chives

Directions:
1. Preheat the air fryer to 370°F. Combine the olive oil, onion, garlic, and sausage in a baking pan and put it in the air basket. Bake for 4-7 minutes or until the onions are crispy but tender and the sausages are hot. Add the stock, vinegar, brown sugar, and cornstarch to the mixture in the pan and stir. Bake for 5 more minutes until hot. Stir the sour cream and yellow mustard into the sauce, add the potatoes, and stir to coat. Cook for another 2-3 minutes or until hot. Serve topped with freshly chopped chives.

Spicy Hoisin Bbq Pork Chops

Servings: 2
Cooking Time: 12 Minutes

Ingredients:
- 3 tablespoons hoisin sauce
- ¼ cup honey
- 1 tablespoon soy sauce
- 3 tablespoons rice vinegar
- 2 tablespoons brown sugar
- 1½ teaspoons grated fresh ginger
- 1 to 2 teaspoons Sriracha sauce, to taste
- 2 to 3 bone-in center cut pork chops, 1-inch thick (about 1¼ pounds)
- chopped scallions, for garnish

Directions:
1. Combine the hoisin sauce, honey, soy sauce, rice vinegar, brown sugar, ginger, and Sriracha sauce in a small saucepan. Whisk the ingredients together and bring the mixture to a boil over medium-high heat on the stovetop. Reduce the heat and simmer the sauce until it has reduced in volume and thickened slightly – about 10 minutes.
2. Preheat the air fryer to 400°F.
3. Place the pork chops into the air fryer basket and pour half the hoisin BBQ sauce over the top. Air-fry for 6 minutes. Then, flip the chops over, pour the remaining hoisin BBQ sauce on top and air-fry for 6 more minutes, depending on the thickness of the pork chops. The internal temperature of the pork chops should be 155°F when tested with an instant read thermometer.
4. Let the pork chops rest for 5 minutes before serving. You can spoon a little of the sauce from the bottom drawer of the air fryer over the top if desired. Sprinkle with chopped scallions and serve.

Zesty London Broil

Servings: 4
Cooking Time: 28 Minutes

Ingredients:
- ⅔ cup ketchup
- ¼ cup honey
- ¼ cup olive oil
- 2 tablespoons apple cider vinegar
- 2 tablespoons Worcestershire sauce
- 2 tablespoons minced onion
- ½ teaspoon paprika
- 1 teaspoon salt
- 1 teaspoon freshly ground black pepper
- 2 pounds London broil, top round or flank steak (about 1-inch thick)

Directions:
1. Combine the ketchup, honey, olive oil, apple cider vinegar, Worcestershire sauce, minced onion, paprika, salt and pepper in a small bowl and whisk together.
2. Generously pierce both sides of the meat with a fork or meat tenderizer and place it in a shallow dish. Pour the marinade mixture over the steak, making sure all sides of the meat get coated with the marinade. Cover and refrigerate overnight.

3. Preheat the air fryer to 400°F.
4. Transfer the London broil to the air fryer basket and air-fry for 28 minutes, depending on how rare or well done you like your steak. Flip the steak over halfway through the cooking time.
5. Remove the London broil from the air fryer and let it rest for five minutes on a cutting board. To serve, thinly slice the meat against the grain and transfer to a serving platter.

Peppered Steak Bites

Servings: 4
Cooking Time: 14 Minutes

Ingredients:
- 1 pound sirloin steak, cut into 1-inch cubes
- ½ teaspoon coarse sea salt
- 1 teaspoon coarse black pepper
- 2 teaspoons Worcestershire sauce
- ½ teaspoon garlic powder
- ¼ teaspoon red pepper flakes
- ¼ cup chopped parsley

Directions:
1. Preheat the air fryer to 390°F.
2. In a large bowl, place the steak cubes and toss with the salt, pepper, Worcestershire sauce, garlic powder, and red pepper flakes.
3. Pour the steak into the air fryer basket and cook for 10 to 14 minutes, depending on how well done you prefer your bites. Starting at the 8-minute mark, toss the steak bites every 2 minutes to check for doneness.
4. When the steak is cooked, remove it from the basket to a serving bowl and top with the chopped parsley. Allow the steak to rest for 5 minutes before serving.

Sriracha Short Ribs

Servings: 4
Cooking Time: 15 Minutes

Ingredients:
- 2 tsp sesame seeds
- 8 pork short ribs
- ½ cup soy sauce
- ¼ cup rice wine vinegar
- ½ cup chopped onion
- 2 garlic cloves, minced
- 1 tbsp sesame oil

- 1 tsp sriracha
- 4 scallions, thinly sliced
- Salt and pepper to taste

Directions:
1. Put short ribs in a resealable bag along with soy sauce, vinegar, onion, garlic, sesame oil, Sriracha, half of the scallions, salt, and pepper. Seal the bag and toss to coat. Refrigerate for one hour.
2. Preheat air fryer to 380°F. Place the short ribs in the air fryer. Bake for 8-10 minutes, flipping once until crisp. When the ribs are done, garnish with remaining scallions and sesame seeds. Serve and enjoy!

Stuffed Pork Chops

Servings: 4
Cooking Time: 12 Minutes

Ingredients:
- 4 boneless pork chops
- ½ teaspoon salt
- ½ teaspoon black pepper
- ¼ teaspoon paprika
- 1 cup frozen spinach, defrosted and squeezed dry
- 2 cloves garlic, minced
- 2 ounces cream cheese
- ¼ cup grated Parmesan cheese
- 1 tablespoon extra-virgin olive oil

Directions:
1. Pat the pork chops with a paper towel. Make a slit in the side of each pork chop to create a pouch.
2. Season the pork chops with the salt, pepper, and paprika.
3. In a small bowl, mix together the spinach, garlic, cream cheese, and Parmesan cheese.
4. Divide the mixture into fourths and stuff the pork chop pouches. Secure the pouches with toothpicks.
5. Preheat the air fryer to 400°F.
6. Place the stuffed pork chops in the air fryer basket and spray liberally with cooking spray. Cook for 6 minutes, flip and coat with more cooking spray, and cook another 6 minutes. Check to make sure the meat is cooked to an internal temperature of 145°F. Cook the pork chops in batches, as needed.

Sirloin Steak Flatbread

Servings: 2
Cooking Time: 40 Minutes

Ingredients:
- 1 premade flatbread dough
- 1 sirloin steak, cubed
- 2 cups breadcrumbs
- 2 eggs, beaten
- Salt and pepper to taste
- 2 tsp onion powder
- 1 tsp garlic powder
- 1 tsp dried thyme
- ½ onion, sliced
- 2 Swiss cheese slices

Directions:
1. Preheat air fryer to 360°F. Place the breadcrumbs, onion powder, garlic powder, thyme, salt, and pepper in a bowl and stir to combine. Add in the steak cubes, coating all sides. Dip into the beaten eggs, then dip again into the crumbs. Lay the coated steak pieces on half of the greased fryer basket. Place the onion slices on the other half of the basket. Air Fry 6 minutes. Turn the onions over and flip the steak pieces. Continue cooking for another 6 minutes. Roll the flatbread out and pierce it several times with a fork. Cover with Swiss cheese slices.
2. When the steak and onions are ready, remove them to the cheese-covered flatbread dough. Fold the flatbread over. Arrange the folded flatbread on the frying basket. Bake for 10 minutes, flipping once until golden brown. Serve.

Chinese-style Lamb Chops

Servings: 4
Cooking Time: 25 Minutes

Ingredients:
- 8 lamb chops, trimmed
- 2 tbsp scallions, sliced
- ¼ tsp Chinese five-spice
- 3 garlic cloves, crushed
- ½ tsp ginger powder
- ¼ cup dark soy sauce
- 2 tsp orange juice
- 3 tbsp honey
- ½ tbsp light brown sugar
- ¼ tsp red pepper flakes

Directions:
1. Season the chops with garlic, ginger, soy sauce, five-spice powder, orange juice, and honey in a bowl. Toss to coat. Cover the bowl with plastic wrap and marinate for 2 hours and up to overnight.
2. Preheat air fryer to 400°F. Remove the chops from the bowl but reserve the marinade. Place the chops in the greased frying basket and Bake for 5 minutes. Using tongs, flip the chops. Brush the lamb with the reserved marinade, then sprinkle with brown sugar and pepper flakes. Cook for another 4 minutes until brown and caramelized medium-rare. Serve with scallions on top.

Peachy Pork Chops

Servings: 2
Cooking Time: 20 Minutes

Ingredients:
- 2 tbsp peach preserves
- 2 tbsp tomato paste
- 1 tbsp Dijon mustard
- 1 tsp BBQ sauce
- 1 tbsp lime juice
- 1 tbsp olive oil
- 2 cloves garlic, minced
- 2 pork chops

Directions:
1. Whisk all ingredients in a bowl until well mixed and let chill covered in the fridge for 30 minutes. Preheat air fryer to 350°F. Place pork chops in the frying basket and Air Fry for 12 minutes or until cooked through and tender. Transfer the chops to a cutting board and let sit for 5 minutes before serving.

Korean-style Lamb Shoulder Chops

Servings: 3
Cooking Time: 28 Minutes

Ingredients:
- ⅓ cup Regular or low-sodium soy sauce or gluten-free tamari sauce
- 1½ tablespoons Toasted sesame oil
- 1½ tablespoons Granulated white sugar
- 2 teaspoons Minced peeled fresh ginger
- 1 teaspoon Minced garlic
- ¼ teaspoon Red pepper flakes
- 3 6-ounce bone-in lamb shoulder chops, any excess fat trimmed
- ⅔ cup Tapioca flour
- Vegetable oil spray

Directions:
1. Put the soy or tamari sauce, sesame oil, sugar, ginger, garlic, and red pepper flakes in a large, heavy zip-closed plastic bag. Add the chops, seal, and rub the marinade evenly over them through the bag. Refrigerate for at least 2 hours or up to 6 hours, turning the bag at least once so the chops move around in the marinade.
2. Set the bag out on the counter as the air fryer heats. Preheat the air fryer to 375°F.
3. Pour the tapioca flour on a dinner plate or in a small pie plate. Remove a chop from the marinade and dredge it on both sides in the tapioca flour, coating it evenly and well. Coat both sides with vegetable oil spray, set it in the basket, and dredge and spray the remaining chop(s), setting them in the basket in a single layer with space between them. Discard the bag with the marinade.
4. Air-fry, turning once, for 25 minutes, or until the chops are well browned and tender when pierced with the point of a paring knife. If the machine is at 360°F, you may need to add up to 3 minutes to the cooking time.
5. Use kitchen tongs to transfer the chops to a wire rack. Cool for just a couple of minutes before serving.

Friday Night Cheeseburgers

Servings: 4
Cooking Time: 20 Minutes

Ingredients:
- 1 lb ground beef
- 1 tsp Worcestershire sauce
- 1 tbsp allspice
- Salt and pepper to taste
- 4 cheddar cheese slices
- 4 buns

Directions:
1. Preheat air fryer to 360°F. Combine beef, Worcestershire sauce, allspice, salt and pepper in a large bowl. Divide into 4 equal portions and shape into patties. Place the burgers in the greased frying basket and Air Fry for 8 minutes. Flip and cook for another 3-4 minutes. Top each burger with cheddar cheese and cook for another minute so the cheese melts. Transfer to a bun and serve.

Taco Pie With Meatballs

Servings: 4
Cooking Time: 40 Minutes + Cooling Time

Ingredients:
- 1 cup shredded quesadilla cheese
- 1 cup shredded Colby cheese
- 10 cooked meatballs, halved
- 1 cup salsa
- 1 cup canned refried beans
- 2 tsp chipotle powder
- ½ tsp ground cumin
- 4 corn tortillas

Directions:
1. Preheat the air fryer to 375°F. Combine the meatball halves, salsa, refried beans, chipotle powder, and cumin in a bowl. In a baking pan, add a tortilla and top with one-quarter of the meatball mixture. Sprinkle one-quarter of the cheeses on top and repeat the layers three more times, ending with cheese. Put the pan in the fryer. Bake for 15-20 minutes until the pie is bubbling and the cheese has melted. Let cool on a wire rack for 10 minutes. Run a knife around the edges of the pan and remove the sides of the pan, then cut into wedges to serve.

Balsamic Marinated Rib Eye Steak With Balsamic Fried Cipollini Onions

Servings: 2
Cooking Time: 22-26 Minutes

Ingredients:
- 3 tablespoons balsamic vinegar
- 2 cloves garlic, sliced
- 1 tablespoon Dijon mustard
- 1 teaspoon fresh thyme leaves
- 1 (16-ounce) boneless rib eye steak
- coarsely ground black pepper
- salt
- 1 (8-ounce) bag cipollini onions, peeled
- 1 teaspoon balsamic vinegar

Directions:
1. Combine the 3 tablespoons of balsamic vinegar, garlic, Dijon mustard and thyme in a small bowl. Pour this marinade over the steak. Pierce the steak several times with a paring knife or
2. a needle-style meat tenderizer and season it generously with coarsely ground black pepper. Flip the steak over and pierce the other side in a similar fashion, seasoning again with the coarsely ground black pepper. Marinate the steak for 2 to 24 hours in the refrigerator. When you are ready to cook, remove the steak from the refrigerator and let it sit at room temperature for 30 minutes.
3. Preheat the air fryer to 400°F.
4. Season the steak with salt and air-fry at 400°F for 12 minutes (medium-rare), 14 minutes (medium), or 16 minutes (well-done), flipping the steak once half way through the cooking time.
5. While the steak is air-frying, toss the onions with 1 teaspoon of balsamic vinegar and season with salt.
6. Remove the steak from the air fryer and let it rest while you fry the onions. Transfer the onions to the air fryer basket and air-fry for 10 minutes, adding a few more minutes if your onions are very large. Then, slice the steak on the bias and serve with the fried onions on top.

Ground Beef Calzones

Servings: 6
Cooking Time: 30 Minutes

Ingredients:
- 1 refrigerated pizza dough
- 1 cup shredded mozzarella
- ½ cup chopped onion
- 2 garlic cloves, minced
- ¼ cup chopped mushrooms
- 1 lb ground beef
- 1 tbsp pizza seasoning
- Salt and pepper to taste
- 1 ½ cups marinara sauce
- 1 tsp flour

Directions:
1. Warm 1 tbsp of oil in a skillet over medium heat. Stir-fry onion, garlic and mushrooms for 2-3 minutes or until aromatic. Add beef, pizza seasoning, salt and pepper. Use a large spoon to break up the beef. Cook for 3 minutes or until brown. Stir in marinara sauce and set aside.
2. On a floured work surface, roll out pizza dough and cut into 6 equal-sized rectangles. On each rectangle, add ½ cup of beef and top with 1 tbsp of shredded cheese. Fold one side of the dough over the filling to the opposite side. Press the edges using the back of a fork to seal them. Preheat air fryer to 400°F. Place the first batch of calzones in the air fryer and spray with cooking oil. Bake for 10 minutes. Let cool slightly and serve warm.

Sweet And Sour Pork

Servings: 2
Cooking Time: 11 Minutes

Ingredients:
- ⅓ cup all-purpose flour
- ⅓ cup cornstarch
- 2 teaspoons Chinese 5-spice powder
- 1 teaspoon salt
- freshly ground black pepper
- 1 egg
- 2 tablespoons milk
- ¾ pound boneless pork, cut into 1-inch cubes
- vegetable or canola oil, in a spray bottle
- 1½ cups large chunks of red and green peppers

- ½ cup ketchup
- 2 tablespoons rice wine vinegar or apple cider vinegar
- 2 tablespoons brown sugar
- ¼ cup orange juice
- 1 tablespoon soy sauce
- 1 clove garlic, minced
- 1 cup cubed pineapple
- chopped scallions

Directions:

1. Set up a dredging station with two bowls. Combine the flour, cornstarch, Chinese 5-spice powder, salt and pepper in one large bowl. Whisk the egg and milk together in a second bowl. Dredge the pork cubes in the flour mixture first, then dip them into the egg and then back into the flour to coat on all sides. Spray the coated pork cubes with vegetable or canola oil.
2. Preheat the air fryer to 400°F.
3. Toss the pepper chunks with a little oil and air-fry at 400°F for 5 minutes, shaking the basket halfway through the cooking time.
4. While the peppers are cooking, start making the sauce. Combine the ketchup, rice wine vinegar, brown sugar, orange juice, soy sauce, and garlic in a medium saucepan and bring the mixture to a boil on the stovetop. Reduce the heat and simmer for 5 minutes. When the peppers have finished air-frying, add them to the saucepan along with the pineapple chunks. Simmer the peppers and pineapple in the sauce for an additional 2 minutes. Set aside and keep warm.
5. Add the dredged pork cubes to the air fryer basket and air-fry at 400°F for 6 minutes, shaking the basket to turn the cubes over for the last minute of the cooking process.
6. When ready to serve, toss the cooked pork with the pineapple, peppers and sauce. Serve over white rice and garnish with chopped scallions.

Pork Chops

Servings: 2
Cooking Time: 16 Minutes

Ingredients:

- 2 bone-in, centercut pork chops, 1-inch thick (10 ounces each)
- 2 teaspoons Worcestershire sauce

- salt and pepper
- cooking spray

Directions:

1. Rub the Worcestershire sauce into both sides of pork chops.
2. Season with salt and pepper to taste.
3. Spray air fryer basket with cooking spray and place the chops in basket side by side.
4. Cook at 360°F for 16 minutes or until well done. Let rest for 5minutes before serving.

Better-than-chinese-take-out Sesame Beef

Servings: 4
Cooking Time: 14 Minutes

Ingredients:

- 1¼ pounds Beef flank steak
- 2½ tablespoons Regular or low-sodium soy sauce or gluten-free tamari sauce
- 2 tablespoons Toasted sesame oil
- 2½ teaspoons Cornstarch
- 1 pound 2 ounces (about 4½ cups) Frozen mixed vegetables for stir-fry, thawed, seasoning packet discarded
- 3 tablespoons Unseasoned rice vinegar (see here)
- 3 tablespoons Thai sweet chili sauce
- 2 tablespoons Light brown sugar
- 2 tablespoons White sesame seeds
- 2 teaspoons Water
- Vegetable oil spray
- 1½ tablespoons Minced peeled fresh ginger
- 1 tablespoon Minced garlic

Directions:

1. Set the flank steak on a cutting board and run your clean fingers across it to figure out which way the meat's fibers are running. (Usually, they run the long way from end to end, or perhaps slightly at an angle lengthwise along the cut.) Cut the flank steak into three pieces parallel to the meat's grain. Then cut each of these pieces into ½-inch-wide strips against the grain.
2. Put the meat strips in a large bowl. For a small batch, add 2 teaspoons of the soy or tamari sauce, 2 teaspoons of the sesame oil, and ½ teaspoon of the cornstarch; for a medium batch, add 1 tablespoon of the soy or tamari sauce, 1 tablespoon of the sesame oil, and 1 teaspoon of

the cornstarch; and for a large batch, add 1½ tablespoons of the soy or tamari sauce, 1½ tablespoons of the sesame oil, and 1½ teaspoons of the cornstarch. Toss well until the meat is thoroughly coated in the marinade. Set aside at room temperature.

3. Preheat the air fryer to 400°F.

4. When the machine is at temperature, place the beef strips in the basket in as close to one layer as possible. The strips will overlap or even cover each other. Air-fry for 10 minutes, tossing and rearranging the strips three times so that the covered parts get exposed, until browned and even a little crisp. Pour the strips into a clean bowl.

5. Spread the vegetables in the basket and air-fry undisturbed for 4 minutes, just until they are heated through and somewhat softened. Pour these into the bowl with the meat strips. Turn off the air fryer.

6. Whisk the rice vinegar, sweet chili sauce, brown sugar, sesame seeds, the remaining soy sauce, and the remaining sesame oil in a small bowl until well combined. For a small batch, whisk the remaining 1 teaspoon cornstarch with the water in a second small bowl to make a smooth slurry; for medium batch, whisk the remaining 1½ teaspoons cornstarch with the water in a second small bowl to make a smooth slurry; and for a large batch, whisk the remaining 2 teaspoons cornstarch with the water in a second small bowl to make a smooth slurry.

7. Generously coat the inside of a large wok with vegetable oil spray, then set the wok over high heat for a few minutes. Add the ginger and garlic; stir-fry for 10 seconds or so, just until fragrant. Add the meat and vegetables; stir-fry for 1 minute to heat through.

8. Add the rice vinegar mixture and continue stir-frying until the sauce is bubbling, less than 1 minute. Add the cornstarch slurry and stir-fry until the sauce has thickened, just a few seconds. Remove the wok from the heat and serve hot.

Asian-style Flank Steak

Servings: 4
Cooking Time: 25 Minutes

Ingredients:
- 1 lb flank steak, cut into strips
- 4 tbsp cornstarch
- Black pepper to taste
- 1 tbsp grated ginger
- 3 garlic cloves, minced
- 2/3 cup beef stock
- 2 tbsp soy sauce
- 2 tbsp light brown sugar
- 2 scallions, chopped
- 1 tbsp sesame seeds

Directions:
1. Preheat the air fryer to 400°F. Sprinkle the beef with 3 tbsp of cornstarch and pepper, then toss to coat. Line the frying basket with round parchment paper with holes poked in it. Add the steak and spray with cooking oil. Bake or 8-12 minutes, shaking after 5 minutes until the beef is browned. Remove from the fryer and set aside. Combine the remaining cornstarch, ginger, garlic, beef stock, soy sauce, sugar, and scallions in a bowl and put it in the frying basket. Bake for 5-8 minutes, stirring after 3 minutes until the sauce is thick and glossy. Plate the beef, pour the sauce over, toss, and sprinkle with sesame seeds to serve.

Poultry Recipes

Poblano Bake..40
Maewoon Chicken Legs...40
Buttermilk-fried Drumsticks 41
Simple Salsa Chicken Thighs 41
Cheesy Chicken Tenders 41
Chicken Wings Al Ajillo..41
Chicago-style Turkey Meatballs 42
Rich Turkey Burgers 42
Hazelnut Chicken Salad With Strawberries 42
Turkey-hummus Wraps...42
Easy Turkey Meatballs...43
Turkey Tenderloin With A Lemon Touch 43
Satay Chicken Skewers 43
Chicken Nuggets..44
Sunday Chicken Skewers 44
Chipotle Chicken Drumsticks 44
Teriyaki Chicken Drumsticks 45
Mexican Turkey Meatloaves 45
Turkey Burgers 45
Favourite Fried Chicken Wings.......................................46
Intense Buffalo Chicken Wings 46
Fennel & Chicken Ratatouille..46
Spicy Black Bean Turkey Burgers With Cumin-avocado
Spread 47
Chicken Souvlaki Gyros..47
Chicken Wellington 48
Air-fried Turkey Breast With Cherry Glaze......................48
Pickle Brined Fried Chicken..49

Poblano Bake

Servings: 4
Cooking Time: 11 Minutes Per Batch

Ingredients:
- 2 large poblano peppers (approx. 5½ inches long excluding stem)
- ¾ pound ground turkey, raw
- ¾ cup cooked brown rice
- 1 teaspoon chile powder
- ½ teaspoon ground cumin
- ½ teaspoon garlic powder
- 4 ounces sharp Cheddar cheese, grated
- 1 8-ounce jar salsa, warmed

Directions:
1. Slice each pepper in half lengthwise so that you have four wide, flat pepper halves.
2. Remove seeds and membrane and discard. Rinse inside and out.
3. In a large bowl, combine turkey, rice, chile powder, cumin, and garlic powder. Mix well.
4. Divide turkey filling into 4 portions and stuff one into each of the 4 pepper halves. Press lightly to pack down.
5. Place 2 pepper halves in air fryer basket and cook at 390°F for 10minutes or until turkey is well done.
6. Top each pepper half with ¼ of the grated cheese. Cook 1 more minute or just until cheese melts.
7. Repeat steps 5 and 6 to cook remaining pepper halves.
8. To serve, place each pepper half on a plate and top with ¼ cup warm salsa.

Maewoon Chicken Legs

Servings: 4
Cooking Time: 30 Minutes + Chilling Time

Ingredients:
- 4 scallions, sliced, whites and greens separated
- ¼ cup tamari
- 2 tbsp sesame oil
- 1 tsp sesame seeds
- ¼ cup honey
- 2 tbsp gochujang
- 2 tbsp ketchup
- 4 cloves garlic, minced
- ½ tsp ground ginger
- Salt and pepper to taste
- 1 tbsp parsley
- 1 ½ lb chicken legs

Directions:
1. Whisk all ingredients, except chicken and scallion greens, in a bowl. Reserve ¼ cup of marinade. Toss chicken legs in the remaining marinade and chill for 30 minutes.
2. Preheat air fryer at 400ºF. Place chicken legs in the greased frying basket and Air Fry for 10 minutes. Turn chicken. Cook for 8 more minutes. Let sit in a serving dish for 5 minutes. Coat the cooked chicken with the reserved marinade and scatter with scallion greens, sesame seeds and parsley to serve.

Buttermilk-fried Drumsticks

Servings: 2
Cooking Time: 25 Minutes

Ingredients:
- 1 egg
- ½ cup buttermilk
- ¾ cup self-rising flour
- ¾ cup seasoned panko breadcrumbs
- 1 teaspoon salt
- ¼ teaspoon ground black pepper (to mix into coating)
- 4 chicken drumsticks, skin on
- oil for misting or cooking spray

Directions:
1. Beat together egg and buttermilk in shallow dish.
2. In a second shallow dish, combine the flour, panko crumbs, salt, and pepper.
3. Sprinkle chicken legs with additional salt and pepper to taste.
4. Dip legs in buttermilk mixture, then roll in panko mixture, pressing in crumbs to make coating stick. Mist with oil or cooking spray.
5. Spray air fryer basket with cooking spray.
6. Cook drumsticks at 360°F for 10minutes. Turn pieces over and cook an additional 10minutes.
7. Turn pieces to check for browning. If you have any white spots that haven't begun to brown, spritz them with oil or cooking spray. Continue cooking for 5 more minutes or until crust is golden brown and juices run clear. Larger, meatier drumsticks will take longer to cook than small ones.

Simple Salsa Chicken Thighs

Servings:2
Cooking Time: 35 Minutes

Ingredients:
- 1 lb boneless, skinless chicken thighs
- 1 cup mild chunky salsa
- ½ tsp taco seasoning
- 2 lime wedges for serving

Directions:
1. Preheat air fryer to 350°F. Add chicken thighs into a baking pan and pour salsa and taco seasoning over. Place the pan in the frying basket and Air Fry for 30 minutes until golden brown.

Serve with lime wedges.

Cheesy Chicken Tenders

Servings: 4
Cooking Time: 25 Minutes

Ingredients:
- 1 cup grated Parmesan cheese
- ¼ cup grated cheddar
- 1 ¼ lb chicken tenders
- 1 egg, beaten
- 2 tbsp milk
- Salt and pepper to taste
- ½ tsp garlic powder
- 1 tsp dried thyme
- ¼ tsp shallot powder

Directions:
1. Preheat the air fryer to 400°F. Stir the egg and milk until combined. Mix the salt, pepper, garlic, thyme, shallot, cheddar cheese, and Parmesan cheese on a plate. Dip the chicken in the egg mix, then in the cheese mix, and press to coat. Lay the tenders in the frying basket in a single layer. Add a raised rack to cook more at one time. Spray all with oil and Bake for 12-16 minutes, flipping once halfway through cooking. Serve hot.

Chicken Wings Al Ajillo

Servings:4
Cooking Time: 35 Minutes

Ingredients:
- 2 lb chicken wings, split at the joint
- 2 tbsp melted butter
- 2 tbsp grated Cotija cheese
- 4 cloves garlic, minced
- ½ tbsp hot paprika
- ¼ tsp salt

Directions:
1. Preheat air fryer to 250°F. Coat the chicken wings with 1 tbsp of butter. Place them in the basket and Air Fry for 12 minutes, tossing once. In another bowl, whisk 1 tbsp of butter, Cotija cheese, garlic, hot paprika, and salt. Reserve. Increase temperature to 400°F. Air Fry wings for 10 more minutes, tossing twice. Transfer them to the bowl with the sauce, and toss to coat. Serve immediately.

Chicago-style Turkey Meatballs

Servings: 6
Cooking Time: 15 Minutes

Ingredients:
- 1 lb ground turkey
- 1 tbsp orange juice
- Salt and pepper to taste
- ½ tsp smoked paprika
- ½ tsp chili powder
- 1 tsp cumin powder
- ¼ red bell pepper, diced
- 1 diced jalapeño pepper
- 2 garlic cloves, minced

Directions:
1. Preheat air fryer to 400°F. Combine all of the ingredients in a large bowl. Shape into meatballs. Transfer the meatballs into the greased frying basket. Air Fry for 4 minutes, then flip the meatballs. Air Fry for another 3 minutes until cooked through. Serve immediately.

Rich Turkey Burgers

Servings: 4
Cooking Time: 30 Minutes

Ingredients:
- 2 tbsp finely grated Emmental
- 1/3 cup minced onions
- ¼ cup grated carrots
- 2 garlic cloves, minced
- 2 tsp olive oil
- 1 tsp dried marjoram
- 1 egg
- 1 lb ground turkey

Directions:
1. Preheat air fryer to 400°F. Mix the onions, carrots, garlic, olive oil, marjoram, Emmental, and egg in a bowl, then add the ground turkey. Use your hands to mix the ingredients together. Form the mixture into 4 patties. Set them in the air fryer and Air Fry for 18-20 minutes, flipping once until cooked through and golden. Serve.

Hazelnut Chicken Salad With Strawberries

Servings:4
Cooking Time: 30 Minutes

Ingredients:
- 2 chicken breasts, cubed
- Salt and pepper to taste
- ¾ cup mayonnaise
- 1 tbsp lime juice
- ½ cup chopped hazelnuts
- ½ cup chopped celery
- ½ cup diced strawberries

Directions:
1. Preheat air fryer to 350ºF. Sprinkle chicken cubes with salt and pepper. Place them in the frying basket and Air Fry for 9 minutes, shaking once. Remove to a bowl and leave it to cool. Add the mayonnaise, lime juice, hazelnuts, celery, and strawberries. Serve.

Turkey-hummus Wraps

Servings: 4
Cooking Time: 7 Minutes Per Batch

Ingredients:
- 4 large whole wheat wraps
- ½ cup hummus
- 16 thin slices deli turkey
- 8 slices provolone cheese
- 1 cup fresh baby spinach (or more to taste)

Directions:
1. To assemble, place 2 tablespoons of hummus on each wrap and spread to within about a half inch from edges. Top with 4 slices of turkey and 2 slices of provolone. Finish with ¼ cup of baby spinach—or pile on as much as you like.
2. Roll up each wrap. You don't need to fold or seal the ends.
3. Place 2 wraps in air fryer basket, seam side down.
4. Cook at 360°F for 4minutes to warm filling and melt cheese. If you like, you can continue cooking for 3 more minutes, until the wrap is slightly crispy.
5. Repeat step 4 to cook remaining wraps.

Easy Turkey Meatballs

Servings: 4
Cooking Time: 20 Minutes

Ingredients:
- 1 lb ground turkey
- ½ celery stalk, chopped
- 1 egg
- ¼ tsp red pepper flakes
- ¼ cup bread crumbs
- Salt and pepper to taste
- ½ tsp garlic powder
- ½ tsp onion powder
- ½ tsp cayenne pepper

Directions:
1. Preheat air fryer to 360°F. Add all of the ingredients to a bowl and mix well. Shape the mixture into 12 balls and arrange them on the greased frying basket. Air Fry for 10-12 minutes or until the meatballs are cooked through and browned. Serve and enjoy!

Turkey Tenderloin With A Lemon Touch

Servings: 4
Cooking Time: 45 Minutes

Ingredients:
- 1 lb boneless, skinless turkey breast tenderloin
- Salt and pepper to taste
- ½ tsp garlic powder
- ½ tsp chili powder
- ½ tsp dried thyme
- 1 lemon, juiced
- 1 tbsp chopped cilantro

Directions:
1. Preheat air fryer to 350°F. Dry the turkey completely with a paper towel, then season with salt, pepper, garlic powder, chili powder, and thyme. Place the turkey in the frying basket. Squeeze the lemon juice over the turkey and bake for 10 minutes. Turn the turkey and bake for another 10 to 15 minutes. Allow to rest for 10 minutes before slicing. Serve sprinkled with cilantro and enjoy.

Satay Chicken Skewers

Servings: 4
Cooking Time: 35 Minutes

Ingredients:
- 2 chicken breasts, cut into strips
- 1 ½ tbsp Thai red curry paste
- ¼ cup peanut butter
- 1 tbsp maple syrup
- 1 tbsp tamari
- 1 tbsp lime juice
- 2 tsp chopped onions
- ¼ tsp minced ginger
- 1 clove garlic, minced
- 1 cup coconut milk
- 1 tsp fish sauce
- 1 tbsp chopped cilantro

Directions:
1. Mix the peanut butter, maple syrup, tamari, lime juice, ¼ tsp of sriracha, onions, ginger, garlic, and 2 tbsp of water in a bowl. Reserve 1 tbsp of the sauce. Set aside. Combine the reserved peanut sauce, fish sauce, coconut milk, Thai red curry paste, cilantro and chicken strips in a bowl and let marinate in the fridge for 15 minutes.
2. Preheat air fryer at 350°F. Thread chicken strips onto skewers and place them on a kebab rack. Place rack in the frying basket and Air Fry for 12 minutes. Serve with previously prepared peanut sauce on the side.

Chicken Nuggets

Servings: 20
Cooking Time: 14 Minutes Per Batch

Ingredients:
- 1 pound boneless, skinless chicken thighs, cut into 1-inch chunks
- ¾ teaspoon salt
- ½ teaspoon black pepper
- ½ teaspoon garlic powder
- ½ teaspoon onion powder
- ½ cup flour
- 2 eggs, beaten
- ½ cup panko breadcrumbs
- 3 tablespoons plain breadcrumbs
- oil for misting or cooking spray

Directions:
1. In the bowl of a food processor, combine chicken, ½ teaspoon salt, pepper, garlic powder, and onion powder. Process in short pulses until chicken is very finely chopped and well blended.
2. Place flour in one shallow dish and beaten eggs in another. In a third dish or plastic bag, mix together the panko crumbs, plain breadcrumbs, and ¼ teaspoon salt.
3. Shape chicken mixture into small nuggets. Dip nuggets in flour, then eggs, then panko crumb mixture.
4. Spray nuggets on both sides with oil or cooking spray and place in air fryer basket in a single layer, close but not overlapping.
5. Cook at 360°F for 10minutes. Spray with oil and cook 4 minutes, until chicken is done and coating is golden brown.
6. Repeat step 5 to cook remaining nuggets.

Sunday Chicken Skewers

Servings: 4
Cooking Time: 25 Minutes

Ingredients:
- 1 green bell pepper, cut into chunks
- 1 red bell pepper, cut into chunks
- 4 chicken breasts, cubed
- 1 tbsp chicken seasoning
- Salt and pepper to taste
- 16 cherry tomatoes
- 8 pearl onions, peeled

Directions:
1. Preheat air fryer to 360°F. Season the cubes with chicken seasoning, salt, and pepper. Thread metal skewers with chicken, bell pepper chunks, cherry tomatoes, and pearl onions. Put the kabobs in the greased frying basket. Bake for 14-16 minutes, flipping once until cooked through. Let cool slightly. Serve.

Chipotle Chicken Drumsticks

Servings: 4
Cooking Time: 40 Minutes

Ingredients:
- 1 can chipotle chilies packed in adobe sauce
- 2 tbsp grated Mexican cheese
- 6 chicken drumsticks
- 1 egg, beaten
- ½ cup bread crumbs
- 1 tbsp corn flakes
- Salt and pepper to taste

Directions:
1. Preheat air fryer to 350°F. Place the chilies in the sauce in your blender and pulse until a fine paste is formed. Transfer to a bowl and add the beaten egg. Combine thoroughly. Mix the breadcrumbs, Mexican cheese, corn flakes, salt, and pepper in a separate bowl, and set aside.
2. Coat the chicken drumsticks with the crumb mixture, then dip into the bowl with wet ingredients, then dip again into the dry ingredients. Arrange the chicken drumsticks on the greased frying basket in a single flat layer. Air Fry for 14-16 minutes, turning each chicken drumstick over once. Serve warm.

Teriyaki Chicken Drumsticks

Servings: 2
Cooking Time: 17 Minutes

Ingredients:

- 2 tablespoons soy sauce*
- ¼ cup dry sherry
- 1 tablespoon brown sugar
- 2 tablespoons water
- 1 tablespoon rice wine vinegar
- 1 clove garlic, crushed
- 1-inch fresh ginger, peeled and sliced
- pinch crushed red pepper flakes
- 4 to 6 bone-in, skin-on chicken drumsticks
- 1 tablespoon cornstarch
- fresh cilantro leaves

Directions:

1. Make the marinade by combining the soy sauce, dry sherry, brown sugar, water, rice vinegar, garlic, ginger and crushed red pepper flakes. Pour the marinade over the chicken legs, cover and let the chicken marinate for 1 to 4 hours in the refrigerator.
2. Preheat the air fryer to 380°F.
3. Transfer the chicken from the marinade to the air fryer basket, transferring any extra marinade to a small saucepan. Air-fry at 380°F for 8 minutes. Flip the chicken over and continue to air-fry for another 6 minutes, watching to make sure it doesn't brown too much.
4. While the chicken is cooking, bring the reserved marinade to a simmer on the stovetop. Dissolve the cornstarch in 2 tablespoons of water and stir this into the saucepan. Bring to a boil to thicken the sauce. Remove the garlic clove and slices of ginger from the sauce and set aside.
5. When the time is up on the air fryer, brush the thickened sauce on the chicken and air-fry for 3 more minutes. Remove the chicken from the air fryer and brush with the remaining sauce.
6. Serve over rice and sprinkle the cilantro leaves on top.

Mexican Turkey Meatloaves

Servings: 4
Cooking Time: 30 Minutes

Ingredients:

- ¼ cup jarred chunky mild salsa
- 1 lb ground turkey
- 1/3 cup bread crumbs
- 1/3 cup canned black beans
- 1/3 cup frozen corn
- ¼ cup minced onion
- ¼ cup chopped scallions
- 2 tbsp chopped cilantro
- 1 egg, beaten
- 1 tbsp tomato puree
- 1 tsp salt
- ½ tsp ground cumin
- 1 tsp Mulato chile powder
- ½ tsp ground aniseed
- ¼ tsp ground cloves
- 2 tbsp ketchup
- 2 tbsp jarred mild salsa

Directions:

1. In a bowl, use your hands to mix the turkey, bread crumbs, beans, corn, salsa, onion, scallions, cilantro, egg, tomato puree, salt, chile powder, aniseed, cloves, and cumin. Shape into 4 patties about 1-inch in thickness.
2. Preheat air fryer to 350°F. Put the meatloaves in the greased frying basket and Bake for about 18-20 minutes, flipping once until cooked through. Stir together the ketchup and salsa in a small bowl. When all loaves are cooked, brush them with the glaze and return to the fryer to heat up for 2 minutes. Serve immediately.

Turkey Burgers

Servings: 4
Cooking Time: 13 Minutes

Ingredients:

- 1 pound ground turkey
- ¼ cup diced red onion
- 1 tablespoon grilled chicken seasoning
- ½ teaspoon dried parsley
- ½ teaspoon salt
- 4 slices provolone cheese
- 4 whole-grain sandwich buns
- Suggested toppings: lettuce, sliced tomatoes,

dill pickles, and mustard

Directions:
1. Combine the turkey, onion, chicken seasoning, parsley, and salt and mix well.
2. Shape into 4 patties.
3. Cook at 360°F for 11 minutes or until turkey is well done and juices run clear.
4. Top each burger with a slice of cheese and cook 2 minutes to melt.
5. Serve on buns with your favorite toppings.

Favourite Fried Chicken Wings

Servings: 4
Cooking Time: 30 Minutes

Ingredients:
- 16 chicken wings
- 1 tsp garlic powder
- ½ tsp paprika
- 1 tsp chicken seasoning
- Black pepper to taste
- ½ cup flour
- ¼ cup sour cream
- 2 tsp red chili flakes

Directions:
1. Preheat air fryer to 400°F. Put the drumettes in a resealable bag along with garlic powder, chicken seasoning, paprika, and pepper. Seal the bag and shake until the chicken is completely coated. Prepare a clean resealable bag and add the flour. Pour sour cream in a large bowl. Dunk the drumettes into the sour cream, then transfer them to the bag of flour. Seal the bag and shake until coated and repeat until all of the wings are coated. Transfer the drumettes to the frying basket. Lightly spray them with cooking oil and Air Fry for 23-25 minutes, shaking the basket a few times until crispy and golden brown. Allow to cool slightly. Sprinkle with red chili flakes and serve.

Intense Buffalo Chicken Wings

Servings: 2
Cooking Time: 40 Minutes

Ingredients:
- 8 chicken wings
- ½ cup melted butter
- 2 tbsp Tabasco sauce
- ½ tbsp lemon juice
- 1 tbsp Worcestershire sauce
- 2 tsp cayenne pepper
- 1 tsp garlic powder
- 1 tsp lemon zest
- Salt and pepper to taste

Directions:
1. Preheat air fryer to 350°F. Place the melted butter, Tabasco, lemon juice, Worcestershire sauce, cayenne, garlic powder, lemon zest, salt, and pepper in a bowl and stir to combine. Dip the chicken wings into the mixture, coating thoroughly. Lay the coated chicken wings on the foil-lined frying basket in an even layer. Air Fry for 16-18 minutes. Shake the basket several times during cooking until the chicken wings are crispy brown. Serve.

Fennel & Chicken Ratatouille

Servings: 4
Cooking Time: 30 Minutes

Ingredients:
- 1 lb boneless, skinless chicken thighs, cubed
- 2 tbsp grated Parmesan cheese
- 1 eggplant, cubed
- 1 zucchini, cubed
- 1 bell pepper, diced
- 1 fennel bulb, sliced
- 1 tsp salt
- 1 tsp Italian seasoning
- 2 tbsp olive oil
- 1 can diced tomatoes
- 1 tsp pasta sauce
- 2 tbsp basil leaves

Directions:
1. Preheat air fryer to 400°F. Mix the chicken, eggplant, zucchini, bell pepper, fennel, salt, Italian seasoning, and oil in a bowl. Place the chicken mixture in the frying basket and Air Fry for 7 minutes. Transfer it to a cake pan. Mix in tomatoes along with juices and pasta sauce. Air Fry for 8 minutes. Scatter with Parmesan and basil. Serve.

Spicy Black Bean Turkey Burgers With Cumin-avocado Spread

Servings: 2
Cooking Time: 20 Minutes

Ingredients:

- 1 cup canned black beans, drained and rinsed
- ¾ pound lean ground turkey
- 2 tablespoons minced red onion
- 1 Jalapeño pepper, seeded and minced
- 2 tablespoons plain breadcrumbs
- ½ teaspoon chili powder
- ¼ teaspoon cayenne pepper
- salt, to taste
- olive or vegetable oil
- 2 slices pepper jack cheese
- toasted burger rolls, sliced tomatoes, lettuce leaves
- Cumin-Avocado Spread:
- 1 ripe avocado
- juice of 1 lime
- 1 teaspoon ground cumin
- ½ teaspoon salt
- 1 tablespoon chopped fresh cilantro
- freshly ground black pepper

Directions:

1. Place the black beans in a large bowl and smash them slightly with the back of a fork. Add the ground turkey, red onion, Jalapeño pepper, breadcrumbs, chili powder and cayenne pepper. Season with salt. Mix with your hands to combine all the ingredients and then shape them into 2 patties. Brush both sides of the burger patties with a little olive or vegetable oil.
2. Preheat the air fryer to 380°F.
3. Transfer the burgers to the air fryer basket and air-fry for 20 minutes, flipping them over halfway through the cooking process. Top the burgers with the pepper jack cheese (securing the slices to the burgers with a toothpick) for the last 2 minutes of the cooking process.
4. While the burgers are cooking, make the cumin avocado spread. Place the avocado, lime juice, cumin and salt in food processor and process until smooth. (For a chunkier spread, you can mash this by hand in a bowl.) Stir in the cilantro and season with freshly ground black pepper. Chill the spread until you are ready to serve.
5. When the burgers have finished cooking, remove them from the air fryer and let them rest on a plate, covered gently with aluminum foil. Brush a little olive oil on the insides of the burger rolls. Place the rolls, cut side up, into the air fryer basket and air-fry at 400°F for 1 minute to toast and warm them.
6. Spread the cumin-avocado spread on the rolls and build your burgers with lettuce and sliced tomatoes and any other ingredient you like. Serve warm with a side of sweet potato fries.

Chicken Souvlaki Gyros

Servings: 4
Cooking Time: 18 Minutes

Ingredients:

- ¼ cup extra-virgin olive oil
- 1 clove garlic, crushed
- 1 tablespoon Italian seasoning
- ½ teaspoon paprika
- ½ lemon, sliced
- ¼ teaspoon salt
- 1 pound boneless, skinless chicken breasts
- 4 whole-grain pita breads
- 1 cup shredded lettuce
- ½ cup chopped tomatoes
- ¼ cup chopped red onion
- ¼ cup cucumber yogurt sauce

Directions:

1. In a large resealable plastic bag, combine the olive oil, garlic, Italian seasoning, paprika, lemon, and salt. Add the chicken to the bag and secure shut. Vigorously shake until all the ingredients are combined. Set in the fridge for 2 hours to marinate.
2. When ready to cook, preheat the air fryer to 360°F.
3. Liberally spray the air fryer basket with olive oil mist. Remove the chicken from the bag and discard the leftover marinade. Place the chicken into the air fryer basket, allowing enough room between the chicken breasts to flip.
4. Cook for 10 minutes, flip, and cook another 8 minutes.
5. Remove the chicken from the air fryer basket when it has cooked (or the internal temperature of the chicken reaches 165°F). Let rest 5 minutes. Then thinly slice the chicken into strips.

6. Assemble the gyros by placing the pita bread on a flat surface and topping with chicken, lettuce, tomatoes, onion, and a drizzle of yogurt sauce.

7. Serve warm.

Chicken Wellington

Servings: 2
Cooking Time: 31 Minutes

Ingredients:
- 2 (5-ounce) boneless, skinless chicken breasts
- ½ cup White Worcestershire sauce
- 3 tablespoons butter
- ½ cup finely diced onion (about ½ onion)
- 8 ounces button mushrooms, finely chopped
- ¼ cup chicken stock
- 2 tablespoons White Worcestershire sauce (or white wine)
- salt and freshly ground black pepper
- 1 tablespoon chopped fresh tarragon
- 2 sheets puff pastry, thawed
- 1 egg, beaten
- vegetable oil

Directions:
1. Place the chicken breasts in a shallow dish. Pour the White Worcestershire sauce over the chicken coating both sides and marinate for 30 minutes.

2. While the chicken is marinating, melt the butter in a large skillet over medium-high heat on the stovetop. Add the onion and sauté for a few minutes, until it starts to soften. Add the mushrooms and sauté for 5 minutes until the vegetables are brown and soft. Deglaze the skillet with the chicken stock, scraping up any bits from the bottom of the pan. Add the White Worcestershire sauce and simmer for 3 minutes until the mixture reduces and starts to thicken. Season with salt and freshly ground black pepper. Remove the mushroom mixture from the heat and stir in the fresh tarragon. Let the mushroom mixture cool.

3. Preheat the air fryer to 360°F.

4. Remove the chicken from the marinade and transfer it to the air fryer basket. Tuck the small end of the chicken breast under the thicker part to shape it into a circle rather than an oval. Pour the marinade over the chicken and air-fry for 10 minutes.

5. Roll out the puff pastry and cut out two 6-inch squares. Brush the perimeter of each square with the egg wash. Place half of the mushroom mixture in the center of each puff pastry square. Place the chicken breasts, top side down on the mushroom mixture. Starting with one corner of puff pastry and working in one direction, pull the pastry up over the chicken to enclose it and press the ends of the pastry together in the middle. Brush the pastry with the egg wash to seal the edges. Turn the Wellingtons over and set aside.

6. To make a decorative design with the remaining puff pastry, cut out four 10-inch strips. For each Wellington, twist two of the strips together, place them over the chicken breast wrapped in puff pastry, and tuck the ends underneath to seal it. Brush the entire top and sides of the Wellingtons with the egg wash.

7. Preheat the air fryer to 350°F.

8. Spray or brush the air fryer basket with vegetable oil. Air-fry the chicken Wellingtons for 13 minutes. Carefully turn the Wellingtons over. Air-fry for another 8 minutes. Transfer to serving plates, light a candle and enjoy!

Air-fried Turkey Breast With Cherry Glaze

Servings: 6
Cooking Time: 54 Minutes

Ingredients:
- 1 (5-pound) turkey breast
- 2 teaspoons olive oil
- 1 teaspoon dried thyme
- ½ teaspoon dried sage
- 1 teaspoon salt
- ½ teaspoon freshly ground black pepper
- ½ cup cherry preserves
- 1 tablespoon chopped fresh thyme leaves
- 1 teaspoon soy sauce*
- freshly ground black pepper

Directions:
1. All turkeys are built differently, so depending on the turkey breast and how your butcher has prepared it, you may need to trim the bottom of the ribs in order to get the turkey to sit upright in the air fryer basket without touching

the heating element. The key to this recipe is getting the right size turkey breast. Once you've managed that, the rest is easy, so make sure your turkey breast fits into the air fryer basket before you Preheat the air fryer.

2. Preheat the air fryer to 350°F.

3. Brush the turkey breast all over with the olive oil. Combine the thyme, sage, salt and pepper and rub the outside of the turkey breast with the spice mixture.

4. Transfer the seasoned turkey breast to the air fryer basket, breast side up, and air-fry at 350°F for 25 minutes. Turn the turkey breast on its side and air-fry for another 12 minutes. Turn the turkey breast on the opposite side and air-fry for 12 more minutes. The internal temperature of the turkey breast should reach 165°F when fully cooked.

5. While the turkey is air-frying, make the glaze by combining the cherry preserves, fresh thyme, soy sauce and pepper in a small bowl. When the cooking time is up, return the turkey breast to an upright position and brush the glaze all over the turkey. Air-fry for a final 5 minutes, until the skin is nicely browned and crispy. Let the turkey rest, loosely tented with foil, for at least 5 minutes before slicing and serving.

Pickle Brined Fried Chicken

Servings: 4
Cooking Time: 47 Minutes

Ingredients:
• 4 bone-in, skin-on chicken legs, cut into drumsticks and thighs (about 3½ pounds)
• pickle juice from a 24-ounce jar of kosher dill pickles
• ½ cup flour
• salt and freshly ground black pepper
• 2 eggs
• 1 cup fine breadcrumbs
• 1 teaspoon salt
• 1 teaspoon freshly ground black pepper
• ½ teaspoon ground paprika
• ⅛ teaspoon ground cayenne pepper
• vegetable or canola oil in a spray bottle

Directions:
1. Place the chicken in a shallow dish and pour the pickle juice over the top. Cover and transfer the chicken to the refrigerator to brine in the pickle juice for 3 to 8 hours.

2. When you are ready to cook, remove the chicken from the refrigerator to let it come to room temperature while you set up a dredging station. Place the flour in a shallow dish and season well with salt and freshly ground black pepper. Whisk the eggs in a second shallow dish. In a third shallow dish, combine the breadcrumbs, salt, pepper, paprika and cayenne pepper.

3. Preheat the air fryer to 370°F.

4. Remove the chicken from the pickle brine and gently dry it with a clean kitchen towel. Dredge each piece of chicken in the flour, then dip it into the egg mixture, and finally press it into the breadcrumb mixture to coat all sides of the chicken. Place the breaded chicken on a plate or baking sheet and spray each piece all over with vegetable oil.

5. Air-fry the chicken in two batches. Place two chicken thighs and two drumsticks into the air fryer basket. Air-fry for 10 minutes. Then, gently turn the chicken pieces over and air-fry for another 10 minutes. Remove the chicken pieces and let them rest on plate – do not cover. Repeat with the second batch of chicken, air-frying for 20 minutes, turning the chicken over halfway through.

6. Lower the temperature of the air fryer to 340°F. Place the first batch of chicken on top of the second batch already in the basket and air-fry for an additional 7 minutes. Serve warm and enjoy.

Vegetable Side Dishes Recipes

Roasted Thyme Asparagus..51
Crispy Cauliflower Puffs..51
Almond Green Beans...51
Buttery Rolls..52
Dijon Artichoke Hearts 52
Sea Salt Radishes 53
Herbed Baby Red Potato Hasselback 53
Simple Roasted Sweet Potatoes 53
Moroccan Cauliflower 53
Panko-crusted Zucchini Fries 54
Buttery Stuffed Tomatoes..54
Baked Shishito Peppers...55
Charred Radicchio Salad 55
Honey-mustard Roasted Cabbage 55
Perfect Broccolini..55
Southern Okra Chips 56
Simple Zucchini Ribbons 56
Roasted Brussels Sprouts 56
Cheese & Bacon Pasta Bake...56
Tomato Candy..57
Veggie Fritters...57
Perfect Broccoli...57
Double Cheese-broccoli Tots 58
Street Corn..58
Grits Again 58
Green Beans..59
Parsnip Fries With Romesco Sauce 59

Roasted Thyme Asparagus

Servings: 4
Cooking Time: 20 Minutes

Ingredients:
- 1 lb asparagus, trimmed
- 2 tsp olive oil
- 3 garlic cloves, minced
- 2 tbsp balsamic vinegar
- ½ tsp dried thyme
- ½ red chili, finely sliced

Directions:
1. Preheat air fryer to 380°F. Put the asparagus and olive oil in a bowl and stir to coat, then put them in the frying basket. Toss some garlic over the asparagus and Roast for 4-8 minutes until crisp-tender. Spritz with balsamic vinegar and toss in some thyme leaves. Top with red chili slices and serve.

Crispy Cauliflower Puffs

Servings: 12
Cooking Time: 9 Minutes

Ingredients:
- 1½ cups Riced cauliflower
- 1 cup (about 4 ounces) Shredded Monterey Jack cheese
- ¾ cup Seasoned Italian-style panko bread crumbs (gluten-free, if a concern)
- 2 tablespoons plus 1 teaspoon All-purpose flour or potato starch
- 2 tablespoons plus 1 teaspoon Vegetable oil
- 1 plus 1 large yolk Large egg(s)
- ¾ teaspoon Table salt
- Vegetable oil spray

Directions:
1. Preheat the air fryer to 375°F.
2. Stir the riced cauliflower, cheese, bread crumbs, flour or potato starch, oil, egg(s) and egg yolk (if necessary), and salt in a large bowl to make a thick batter.
3. Using 2 tablespoons of the batter, form a compact ball between your clean, dry palms. Set it aside and continue forming more balls: 7 more for a small batch, 11 more for a medium batch, or 15 more for a large batch.
4. Generously coat the balls on all sides with vegetable oil spray. Set them in the basket with as much air space between them as possible. Air-fry undisturbed for 7 minutes, or until golden brown and crisp. If the machine is at 360°F, you may need to add 2 minutes to the cooking time.
5. Gently pour the contents of the basket onto a wire rack. Cool the puffs for 5 minutes before serving.

Almond Green Beans

Servings: 4
Cooking Time: 20 Minutes

Ingredients:
- 2 cups green beans, trimmed
- ¼ cup slivered almonds
- 2 tbsp butter, melted
- Salt and pepper to taste
- 2 tsp lemon juice
- Lemon zest and slices

Directions:
1. Preheat air fryer at 375°F. Add almonds to the frying basket and Air Fry for 2 minutes, tossing once. Set aside in a small bowl. Combine the remaining ingredients, except 1 tbsp of butter, in a bowl.
2. Place green beans in the frying basket and Air Fry for 10 minutes, tossing once. Then, transfer them to a large serving dish. Scatter with the melted butter, lemon juice and roasted almonds and toss. Serve immediately garnished with lemon zest and lemon slices.

Buttery Rolls

Servings: 6
Cooking Time: 14 Minutes

Ingredients:

- 6½ tablespoons Room-temperature whole or low-fat milk
- 3 tablespoons plus 1 teaspoon Butter, melted and cooled
- 3 tablespoons plus 1 teaspoon (or 1 medium egg, well beaten) Pasteurized egg substitute, such as Egg Beaters
- 1½ tablespoons Granulated white sugar
- 1¼ teaspoons Instant yeast
- ¼ teaspoon Table salt
- 2 cups, plus more for dusting All-purpose flour
- Vegetable oil
- Additional melted butter, for brushing

Directions:

1. Stir the milk, melted butter, pasteurized egg substitute (or whole egg), sugar, yeast, and salt in a medium bowl to combine. Stir in the flour just until the mixture makes a soft dough.
2. Lightly flour a clean, dry work surface. Turn the dough out onto the work surface. Knead the dough for 5 minutes to develop the gluten.
3. Lightly oil the inside of a clean medium bowl. Gather the dough into a compact ball and set it in the bowl. Turn the dough over so that its surface has oil on it all over. Cover the bowl tightly with plastic wrap and set aside in a warm, draft-free place until the dough has doubled in bulk, about 1½ hours.
4. Punch down the dough, then turn it out onto a clean, dry work surface. Divide it into 5 even balls for a small batch, 6 balls for a medium batch, or 8 balls for a large one.
5. For a small batch, lightly oil the inside of a 6-inch round cake pan and set the balls around its perimeter, separating them as much as possible.
6. For a medium batch, lightly oil the inside of a 7-inch round cake pan and set the balls in it with one ball at its center, separating them as much as possible.
7. For a large batch, lightly oil the inside of an 8-inch round cake pan and set the balls in it with one at the center, separating them as much as possible.
8. Cover with plastic wrap and set aside to rise for 30 minutes.
9. Preheat the air fryer to 350°F.
10. Uncover the pan and brush the rolls with a little melted butter, perhaps ½ teaspoon per roll. When the machine is at temperature, set the cake pan in the basket. Air-fry undisturbed for 14 minutes, or until the rolls have risen and browned.
11. Using kitchen tongs and a nonstick-safe spatula, two hot pads, or silicone baking mitts, transfer the cake pan from the basket to a wire rack. Cool the rolls in the pan for a minute or two. Turn the rolls out onto a wire rack, set them top side up again, and cool for at least another couple of minutes before serving warm.

Dijon Artichoke Hearts

Servings: 4
Cooking Time: 25 Minutes

Ingredients:

- 1 jar artichoke hearts in water, drained
- 1 egg
- 1 tbsp Dijon mustard
- ½ cup bread crumbs
- ¼ cup flour
- 6 basil leaves

Directions:

1. Preheat air fryer to 350ºF. Beat egg and mustard in a bowl. In another bowl, combine bread crumbs and flour. Dip artichoke hearts in egg mixture, then dredge in crumb mixture. Place artichoke hearts in the greased frying basket and Air Fry for 7-10 minutes until crispy. Serve topped with basil. Enjoy!

Sea Salt Radishes

Servings: 4
Cooking Time: 25 Minutes

Ingredients:

- 1 lb radishes
- 2 tbsp olive oil
- ½ tsp sea salt
- ½ tsp garlic powder

Directions:

1. Preheat air fryer to 360°F. Toss the radishes with olive oil, garlic powder, and salt in a bowl. Pour them into the air fryer. Air Fry for 18 minutes, turning once. Serve.

Herbed Baby Red Potato Hasselback

Servings: 4
Cooking Time: 35 Minutes

Ingredients:

- 6 baby red potatoes, scrubbed
- 3 tsp shredded cheddar cheese
- 1 tbsp olive oil
- 2 tbsp butter, melted
- 1 tbsp chopped thyme
- Salt and pepper to taste
- 3 tsp sour cream
- ¼ cup chopped parsley

Directions:

1. Preheat air fryer at 350°F. Make slices in the width of each potato about ¼-inch apart without cutting through. Rub potato slices with olive oil, both outside and in between slices. Place potatoes in the frying basket and Air Fry for 20 minutes, tossing once, brush with melted butter, and scatter with thyme. Remove them to a large serving dish. Sprinkle with salt, black pepper and top with a dollop of cheddar cheese, sour cream. Scatter with parsley to serve.

Simple Roasted Sweet Potatoes

Servings: 2
Cooking Time: 45 Minutes

Ingredients:

- 2 10- to 12-ounce sweet potato(es)

Directions:

1. Preheat the air fryer to 350°F .
2. Prick the sweet potato(es) in four or five different places with the tines of a flatware fork (not in a line but all around).
3. When the machine is at temperature, set the sweet potato(es) in the basket with as much air space between them as possible. Air-fry undisturbed for 45 minutes, or until soft when pricked with a fork.
4. Use kitchen tongs to transfer the sweet potato(es) to a wire rack. Cool for 5 minutes before serving.

Moroccan Cauliflower

Servings: 6
Cooking Time: 15 Minutes

Ingredients:

- 1 tablespoon curry powder
- 2 teaspoons smoky paprika
- ½ teaspoon ground cumin
- ½ teaspoon salt
- 1 head cauliflower, cut into bite-size pieces
- ¼ cup red wine vinegar
- 2 tablespoons extra-virgin olive oil
- 2 tablespoons chopped parsley

Directions:

1. Preheat the air fryer to 370°F.
2. In a large bowl, mix the curry powder, paprika, cumin, and salt. Add the cauliflower and stir to coat. Pour the red wine vinegar over the top and continue stirring.
3. Place the cauliflower into the air fryer basket; drizzle olive oil over the top.
4. Cook the cauliflower for 5 minutes, toss, and cook another 5 minutes. Raise the temperature to 400°F and continue cooking for 4 to 6 minutes, or until crispy.

Panko-crusted Zucchini Fries

Servings: 6
Cooking Time: 8 Minutes

Ingredients:
- 3 medium zucchinis
- ½ cup flour
- 1 teaspoon salt, divided
- ½ teaspoon black pepper, divided
- ¾ teaspoon dried thyme, divided
- 2 large eggs
- 1 ½ cups whole-wheat or plain panko bread-crumbs
- ½ cup grated Parmesan cheese

Directions:
1. Preheat the air fryer to 380°F.
2. Slice the zucchinis in half lengthwise, then into long strips about ½-inch thick, like thick fries.
3. In a medium bowl, mix the flour, ½ teaspoon of the salt, ¼ teaspoon of the black pepper, and ½ teaspoon of thyme.
4. In a separate bowl, whisk together the eggs, ½ teaspoon of the salt, and ¼ teaspoon of the black pepper.
5. In a third bowl, combine the breadcrumbs, cheese, and the remaining ¼ teaspoon of dried thyme.
6. Working with one zucchini fry at a time, dip the zucchini fry first into the flour mixture, then into the whisked eggs, and finally into the breading. Repeat until all the fries are breaded.
7. Place the zucchini fries into the air fryer basket, spray with cooking spray, and cook for 4 minutes; shake the basket and cook another 4 to 6 minutes or until golden brown and crispy.
8. Remove and serve warm.

Buttery Stuffed Tomatoes

Servings: 6
Cooking Time: 15 Minutes

Ingredients:
- 3 8-ounce round tomatoes
- ½ cup plus 1 tablespoon Plain panko bread crumbs (gluten-free, if a concern)
- 3 tablespoons (about ½ ounce) Finely grated Parmesan cheese
- 3 tablespoons Butter, melted and cooled
- 4 teaspoons Stemmed and chopped fresh parsley leaves
- 1 teaspoon Minced garlic
- ¼ teaspoon Table salt
- Up to ¼ teaspoon Red pepper flakes
- Olive oil spray

Directions:
1. Preheat the air fryer to 375°F .
2. Cut the tomatoes in half through their "equators" (that is, not through the stem ends). One at a time, gently squeeze the tomato halves over a trash can, using a clean finger to gently force out the seeds and most of the juice inside, working carefully so that the tomato doesn't lose its round shape or get crushed.
3. Stir the bread crumbs, cheese, butter, parsley, garlic, salt, and red pepper flakes in a bowl until the bread crumbs are moistened and the parsley is uniform throughout the mixture. Pile this mixture into the spaces left in the tomato halves. Press gently to compact the filling. Coat the tops of the tomatoes with olive oil spray.
4. Place the tomatoes cut side up in the basket. They may touch each other. Air-fry for 15 minutes, or until the filling is lightly browned and crunchy.
5. Use nonstick-safe spatula and kitchen tongs for balance to gently transfer the stuffed tomatoes to a platter or a cutting board. Cool for a couple of minutes before serving.

Baked Shishito Peppers

Servings: 2
Cooking Time: 15 Minutes

Ingredients:
- 6 oz shishito peppers
- 1 tsp olive oil
- 1 tsp salt
- ¼ cup soy sauce

Directions:
1. Preheat air fryer at 375°F. Combine all ingredients in a bowl. Place peppers in the frying basket and Bake for 8 minutes until the peppers are blistered, shaking once. Serve with soy sauce for dipping.

Charred Radicchio Salad

Servings: 4
Cooking Time: 5 Minutes

Ingredients:
- 2 Small 5- to 6-ounce radicchio head(s)
- 3 tablespoons Olive oil
- ½ teaspoon Table salt
- 2 tablespoons Balsamic vinegar
- Up to ¼ teaspoon Red pepper flakes

Directions:
1. Preheat the air fryer to 375°F.
2. Cut the radicchio head(s) into quarters through the stem end. Brush the oil over the heads, particularly getting it between the leaves along the cut sides. Sprinkle the radicchio quarters with the salt.
3. When the machine is at temperature, set the quarters cut sides up in the basket with as much air space between them as possible. They should not touch. Air-fry undisturbed for 5 minutes, watching carefully because they burn quickly, until blackened in bits and soft.
4. Use a nonstick-safe spatula to transfer the quarters to a cutting board. Cool for a minute or two, then cut out the thick stems inside the heads. Discard these tough bits and chop the remaining heads into bite-size bits. Scrape them into a bowl. Add the vinegar and red pepper flakes. Toss well and serve warm.

Honey-mustard Roasted Cabbage

Servings: 4
Cooking Time: 35 Minutes

Ingredients:
- 4 cups chopped green cabbage
- 1/3 cup honey mustard dressing
- 1 shallot, chopped
- 2 garlic cloves, minced
- 2 tbsp olive oil
- 1 tbsp lemon juice
- 1 tbsp cornstarch
- ½ tsp fennel seeds

Directions:
1. Preheat the air fryer to 370°F. Toss the cabbage, shallot, olive oil and garlic in a cake pan. Bake for 10 minutes or until the cabbage is wilted, then drain the excess liquid. While the cabbage is cooking, combine the salad dressing, lemon juice, cornstarch, and fennel seeds in a bowl. Take cake pan out of the fryer and pour out any excess liquid. Pour the dressing mix over the drained cabbage and mix well. Return the pan to the fryer and Bake for 7-11 minutes more, stirring twice during cooking until the cabbage is tender and the sauce has thickened. Serve warm.

Perfect Broccolini

Servings: 4
Cooking Time: 15 Minutes

Ingredients:
- 1 pound Broccolini
- Olive oil spray
- Coarse sea salt or kosher salt

Directions:
1. Preheat the air fryer to 375°F.
2. Place the broccolini on a cutting board. Generously coat it with olive oil spray, turning the vegetables and rearranging them before spraying a couple of times more, to make sure everything's well coated, even the flowery bits in their heads.
3. When the machine is at temperature, pile the broccolini in the basket, spreading it into as close to one layer as you can. Air-fry for 5 minutes, tossing once to get any covered or touching parts exposed to the air currents, until the

leaves begin to get brown and even crisp. Watch carefully and use this visual cue to know the moment to stop the cooking.

4. Transfer the broccolini to a platter. Spread out the pieces and sprinkle them with salt to taste.

Southern Okra Chips

Servings: 2
Cooking Time: 20 Minutes

Ingredients:
- 2 eggs
- ¼ cup whole milk
- ¼ cup bread crumbs
- ¼ cup cornmeal
- 1 tbsp Cajun seasoning
- Salt and pepper to taste
- ⅛ tsp chili pepper
- ½ lb okra, sliced
- 1 tbsp butter, melted

Directions:
1. Preheat air fryer at 400°F. Beat the eggs and milk in a bowl. In another bowl, combine the remaining ingredients, except okra and butter. Dip okra chips in the egg mixture, then dredge them in the breadcrumbs mixture. Place okra chips in the greased frying basket and Roast for 7 minutes, shake once and brush with melted butter. Serve right away.

Simple Zucchini Ribbons

Servings: 4
Cooking Time: 15 Minutes

Ingredients:
- 2 zucchini
- 2 tsp butter, melted
- ¼ tsp garlic powder
- ¼ tsp chili flakes
- 8 cherry tomatoes, halved
- Salt and pepper to taste

Directions:
1. Preheat air fryer to 275°F. Cut the zucchini into ribbons with a vegetable peeler. Mix them with butter, garlic, chili flakes, salt, and pepper in a bowl. Transfer to the frying basket and Air Fry for 2 minutes. Toss and add the cherry tomatoes. Cook for another 2 minutes. Serve.

Roasted Brussels Sprouts

Servings: 4
Cooking Time: 25 Minutes

Ingredients:
- ½ cup balsamic vinegar
- 2 tablespoons honey
- 1 pound Brussels sprouts, halved lengthwise
- 2 slices bacon, chopped
- ½ teaspoon garlic powder
- 1 teaspoon salt
- 1 tablespoon extra-virgin olive oil
- ¼ cup grated Parmesan cheese

Directions:
1. Preheat the air fryer to 370°F.
2. In a small saucepan, heat the vinegar and honey for 8 to 10 minutes over medium-low heat, or until the balsamic vinegar reduces by half to create a thick balsamic glazing sauce.
3. While the balsamic glaze is reducing, in a large bowl, toss together the Brussels sprouts, bacon, garlic powder, salt, and olive oil. Pour the mixture into the air fryer basket and cook for 10 minutes; check for doneness. Cook another 2 to 5 minutes or until slightly crispy and tender.
4. Pour the balsamic glaze into a serving bowl and add the cooked Brussels sprouts to the dish, stirring to coat. Top with grated Parmesan cheese and serve.

Cheese & Bacon Pasta Bake

Servings: 4
Cooking Time: 35 Minutes

Ingredients:
- ½ cup shredded sharp cheddar cheese
- ½ cup shredded mozzarella cheese
- 4 oz cooked bacon, crumbled
- 3 tbsp butter, divided
- 1 tbsp flour
- 1 tsp black pepper
- 2 oz crushed feta cheese
- ¼ cup heavy cream
- ½ lb cooked rotini
- ¼ cup bread crumbs

Directions:
1. Melt 2 tbsp of butter in a skillet over medium heat. Stir in flour until the sauce thickens. Stir in

all cheeses, black pepper and heavy cream and cook for 2 minutes until creamy. Toss in rotini and bacon until well coated. Spoon rotini mixture into a greased cake pan.

2. Preheat air fryer at 370°F. Microwave the remaining butter in 10-seconds intervals until melted. Then stir in breadcrumbs. Scatter over pasta mixture. Place cake pan in the frying basket and Bake for 15 minutes. Let sit for 10 minutes before serving.

Tomato Candy

Servings: 12
Cooking Time: 120 Minutes

Ingredients:
- 6 Small Roma or plum tomatoes, halved lengthwise
- 1½ teaspoons Coarse sea salt or kosher salt

Directions:
1. Before you turn the machine on, set the tomatoes cut side up in a single layer in the basket (or the basket attachment). They can touch each other, but try to leave at least a fraction of an inch between them (depending, of course, on the size of the basket or basket attachment). Sprinkle the cut sides of the tomatoes with the salt.
2. Set the machine to cook at 225°F (or 230°F, if that's the closest setting). Put the basket in the machine and air-fry for 2 hours, or until the tomatoes are dry but pliable, with a little moisture down in their centers.
3. Remove the basket from the machine and cool the tomatoes in it for 10 minutes before gently transferring them to a plate for serving, or to a shallow dish that you can cover and store in the refrigerator for up to 1 week.

Veggie Fritters

Servings: 4
Cooking Time: 35 Minutes

Ingredients:
- ¼ cup crumbled feta cheese
- 1 grated zucchini
- ¼ cup Parmesan cheese
- 2 tbsp minced onion
- 1 tbs powder garlic
- 1 tbsp flour
- 1 tbsp cornmeal
- 1 tbsp butter, melted
- 1 egg
- 2 tsp chopped dill
- 2 tsp chopped parsley
- Salt and pepper to taste
- 1 cup bread crumbs

Directions:
1. Preheat air fryer at 350°F. Squeeze grated zucchini between paper towels to remove excess moisture. In a bowl, combine all ingredients except breadcrumbs. Form mixture into 12 balls, about 2 tbsp each. In a shallow bowl, add breadcrumbs. Roll each ball in breadcrumbs, covering all sides. Place fritters on an ungreased pizza pan. Place in the frying basket and Air Fry for 11 minutes, flipping once. Serve.

Perfect Broccoli

Servings: 4
Cooking Time: 12 Minutes

Ingredients:
- 5 cups (about 1 pound 10 ounces) 1- to 1½-inch fresh broccoli florets (not frozen)
- Olive oil spray
- ¾ teaspoon Table salt

Directions:
1. Preheat the air fryer to 375°F .
2. Put the broccoli florets in a big bowl, coat them generously with olive oil spray, then toss to coat all surfaces, even down into the crannies, spraying them in a couple of times more. Sprinkle the salt on top and toss again.
3. When the machine is at temperature, pour the florets into the basket. Air-fry for 10 minutes, tossing and rearranging the pieces twice so that all the covered or touching bits are eventually exposed to the air currents, until lightly browned but still crunchy. (If the machine is at 360°F, you may have to add 2 minutes to the cooking time.)
4. Pour the florets into a serving bowl. Cool for a minute or two, then serve hot.

Double Cheese-broccoli Tots

Servings:4
Cooking Time: 30 Minutes

Ingredients:
- 1/3 cup grated sharp cheddar cheese
- 1 cup riced broccoli
- 1 egg
- 1 oz herbed Boursin cheese
- 1 tbsp grated onion
- 1/3 cup bread crumbs
- ½ tsp salt
- ¼ tsp garlic powder

Directions:
1. Preheat air fryer to 375ºF. Mix the riced broccoli, egg, cheddar cheese, Boursin cheese, onion, bread crumbs, salt, and garlic powder in a bowl. Form into 12 rectangular mounds. Cut a piece of parchment paper to fit the bottom of the frying basket, place the tots, and Air Fry for 9 minutes. Let chill for 5 minutes before serving.

Street Corn

Servings: 4
Cooking Time: 10 Minutes

Ingredients:
- 1 tablespoon butter
- 4 ears corn
- ⅓ cup plain Greek yogurt
- 2 tablespoons Parmesan cheese
- ½ teaspoon paprika
- ½ teaspoon garlic powder
- ¼ teaspoon salt
- ¼ teaspoon black pepper
- ¼ cup finely chopped cilantro

Directions:
1. Preheat the air fryer to 400°F.
2. In a medium microwave-safe bowl, melt the butter in the microwave. Lightly brush the outside of the ears of corn with the melted butter.
3. Place the corn into the air fryer basket and cook for 5 minutes, flip the corn, and cook another 5 minutes.
4. Meanwhile, in a medium bowl, mix the yogurt, cheese, paprika, garlic powder, salt, and pepper. Set aside.
5. Carefully remove the corn from the air fryer and let cool 3 minutes. Brush the outside edg-

es with the yogurt mixture and top with fresh chopped cilantro. Serve immediately.

Grits Again

Servings: 2
Cooking Time: 10 Minutes

Ingredients:
- cooked grits
- plain breadcrumbs
- oil for misting or cooking spray
- honey or maple syrup for serving (optional)

Directions:
1. While grits are still warm, spread them into a square or rectangular baking pan, about ½-inch thick. If your grits are thicker than that, scoop some out into another pan.
2. Chill several hours or overnight, until grits are cold and firm.
3. When ready to cook, pour off any water that has collected in pan and cut grits into 2- to 3-inch squares.
4. Dip grits squares in breadcrumbs and place in air fryer basket in single layer, close but not touching.
5. Cook at 390°F for 10 minutes, until heated through and crispy brown on the outside.
6. Serve while hot either plain or with a drizzle of honey or maple syrup.

Green Beans

Servings: 4
Cooking Time: 12 Minutes

Ingredients:

- 1 pound fresh green beans
- 2 tablespoons Italian salad dressing
- salt and pepper

Directions:

1. Wash beans and snap off stem ends.
2. In a large bowl, toss beans with Italian dressing.
3. Cook at 330°F for 5minutes. Shake basket or stir and cook 5minutes longer. Shake basket again and, if needed, continue cooking for 2 minutes, until as tender as you like. Beans should shrivel slightly and brown in places.
4. Sprinkle with salt and pepper to taste.

Parsnip Fries With Romesco Sauce

Servings: 2
Cooking Time: 24 Minutes

Ingredients:

- Romesco Sauce:
- 1 red bell pepper, halved and seeded
- 1 (1-inch) thick slice of Italian bread, torn into pieces (about 1 to 1½ cups)
- 1 cup almonds, toasted
- olive oil
- ½ Jalapeño pepper, seeded
- 1 tablespoon fresh parsley leaves
- 1 clove garlic
- 2 Roma tomatoes, peeled and seeded (or ⅓ cup canned crushed tomatoes)
- 1 tablespoon red wine vinegar
- ¼ teaspoon smoked paprika
- ½ teaspoon salt
- ¾ cup olive oil
- 3 parsnips, peeled and cut into long strips
- 2 teaspoons olive oil
- salt and freshly ground black pepper

Directions:

1. Preheat the air fryer to 400°F.
2. Place the red pepper halves, cut side down, in the air fryer basket and air-fry for 10 minutes, or until the skin turns black all over. Remove the pepper from the air fryer and let it cool. When it is cool enough to handle, peel the pepper.
3. Toss the torn bread and almonds with a little olive oil and air-fry for 4 minutes, shaking the basket a couple times throughout the cooking time. When the bread and almonds are nicely toasted, remove them from the air fryer and let them cool for just a minute or two.
4. Combine the toasted bread, almonds, roasted red pepper, Jalapeño pepper, parsley, garlic, tomatoes, vinegar, smoked paprika and salt in a food processor or blender. Process until smooth. With the processor running, add the olive oil through the feed tube until the sauce comes together in a smooth paste that is barely pourable.
5. Toss the parsnip strips with the olive oil, salt and freshly ground black pepper and air-fry at 400°F for 10 minutes, shaking the basket a couple times during the cooking process so they brown and cook evenly. Serve the parsnip fries warm with the Romesco sauce to dip into.

Vegetarians Recipes

Roasted Vegetable Stromboli 61
Kale & Lentils With Crispy Onions 61
Mushroom-rice Stuffed Bell Peppers 62
Parmesan Portobello Mushroom Caps......................62
Falafel 62
Bite-sized Blooming Onions...63
Meatless Kimchi Bowls 63
Italian Stuffed Bell Peppers...63
Chicano Rice Bowls 64
Berbere Eggplant Dip..64
Cheddar-bean Flautas 64
Golden Fried Tofu 65
Caprese-style Sandwiches 65
Sesame Orange Tofu With Snow Peas.......................65
Golden Breaded Mushrooms..66
Quinoa Burgers With Feta Cheese And Dill...............66
Vegan French Toast 67
Cheddar Bean Taquitos 67
Pizza Portobello Mushrooms 67
Green Bean & Baby Potato Mix 68
Asparagus, Mushroom And Cheese Soufflés 68
Vegetarian Shepherd´s Pie...68
Fried Rice With Curried Tofu 69
Sweet Roasted Carrots...69
Vegetarian Stuffed Bell Peppers 69
Lentil Fritters 70
Pine Nut Eggplant Dip..70

Roasted Vegetable Stromboli

Servings: 2
Cooking Time: 29 Minutes

Ingredients:
- ½ onion, thinly sliced
- ½ red pepper, julienned
- ½ yellow pepper, julienned
- olive oil
- 1 small zucchini, thinly sliced
- 1 cup thinly sliced mushrooms
- 1½ cups chopped broccoli
- 1 teaspoon Italian seasoning
- salt and freshly ground black pepper
- ½ recipe of Blue Jean Chef Pizza dough (page 231) OR 1 (14-ounce) tube refrigerated pizza dough
- 2 cups grated mozzarella cheese
- ¼ cup grated Parmesan cheese
- ½ cup sliced black olives, optional
- dried oregano
- pizza or marinara sauce

Directions:
1. Preheat the air fryer to 400°F.
2. Toss the onions and peppers with a little olive oil and air-fry the vegetables for 7 minutes, shaking the basket once or twice while the vegetables cook. Add the zucchini, mushrooms, broccoli and Italian seasoning to the basket. Add a little more olive oil and season with salt and freshly ground black pepper. Air-fry for an additional 7 minutes, shaking the basket halfway through. Let the vegetables cool slightly while you roll out the pizza dough.
3. On a lightly floured surface, roll or press the pizza dough out into a 13-inch by 11-inch rectangle, with the long side closest to you. Sprinkle half of the mozzarella and Parmesan cheeses over the dough leaving an empty 1-inch border from the edge farthest away from you. Spoon the roasted vegetables over the cheese, sprinkle the olives over everything and top with the remaining cheese.
4. Start rolling the stromboli away from you and toward the empty border. Make sure the filling stays tightly tucked inside the roll. Finally, tuck the ends of the dough in and pinch the seam shut. Place the seam side down and shape the stromboli into a U-shape to fit into the air fryer basket. Cut 4 small slits with the tip of a sharp knife evenly in the top of the dough, lightly brush the stromboli with a little oil and sprinkle with some dried oregano.
5. Preheat the air fryer to 360°F.
6. Spray or brush the air fryer basket with oil and transfer the U-shaped stromboli to the air fryer basket. Air-fry for 15 minutes, flipping the stromboli over after the first 10 minutes. (Use a plate to invert the Stromboli out of the air fryer basket and then slide it back into the basket off the plate.)
7. To remove, carefully flip the stromboli over onto a cutting board. Let it rest for a couple of minutes before serving. Cut it into 2-inch slices and serve with pizza or marinara sauce.

Kale & Lentils With Crispy Onions

Servings: 4
Cooking Time: 40 Minutes

Ingredients:
- 2 cups cooked red lentils
- 1 onion, cut into rings
- ½ cup kale, steamed
- 3 garlic cloves, minced
- ½ lemon, juiced and zested
- 2 tsp cornstarch
- 1 tsp dried oregano
- Salt and pepper to taste

Directions:
1. Preheat air fryer to 390°F. Put the onion rings in the greased frying basket; do not overlap. Spray with oil and season with salt. Air Fry for 14-16 minutes, stirring twice until crispy and crunchy. Place the kale and lentils into a pan over medium heat and stir until heated through. Remove and add the garlic, lemon juice, corn-

starch, salt, zest, oregano and black pepper. Stir well and pour in bowls. Top with the crisp onion rings and serve.

Mushroom-rice Stuffed Bell Peppers

Servings: 4
Cooking Time: 30 Minutes

Ingredients:
- 4 red bell peppers, tops sliced
- 1 ½ cups cooked rice
- ¼ cup chopped leeks
- ¼ cup sliced mushrooms
- ¾ cup tomato sauce
- Salt and pepper to taste
- ¾ cup shredded mozzarella
- 2 tbsp parsley, chopped

Directions:
1. Fill a large pot of water and heat on high until it boils. Remove seeds and membranes from the peppers. Carefully place peppers into the boiling water for 5 minutes. Remove and set aside to cool. Mix together rice, leeks, mushrooms, tomato sauce, parsley, salt, and pepper in a large bowl. Stuff each pepper with the rice mixture. Top with mozzarella.
2. Preheat air fryer to 350°F. Arrange the peppers on the greased frying basket and Bake for 10 minutes. Serve.

Parmesan Portobello Mushroom Caps

Servings: 2
Cooking Time: 14 Minutes

Ingredients:
- ¼ cup flour*
- 1 egg, lightly beaten
- 1 cup seasoned breadcrumbs*
- 2 large portobello mushroom caps, stems and gills removed
- olive oil, in a spray bottle
- ½ cup tomato sauce
- ¾ cup grated mozzarella cheese
- 1 tablespoon grated Parmesan cheese
- 1 tablespoon chopped fresh basil or parsley

Directions:

1. Set up a dredging station with three shallow dishes. Place the flour in the first shallow dish, egg in the second dish and breadcrumbs in the last dish. Dredge the mushrooms in flour, then dip them into the egg and finally press them into the breadcrumbs to coat on all sides. Spray both sides of the coated mushrooms with olive oil.
2. Preheat the air fryer to 400°F.
3. Air-fry the mushrooms at 400°F for 10 minutes, turning them over halfway through the cooking process.
4. Fill the underside of the mushrooms with the tomato sauce and then top the sauce with the mozzarella and Parmesan cheeses. Reset the air fryer temperature to 350°F and air-fry for an additional 4 minutes, until the cheese has melted and is slightly browned.
5. Serve the mushrooms with pasta tossed with tomato sauce and garnish with some chopped fresh basil or parsley.

Falafel

Servings: 4
Cooking Time: 10 Minutes

Ingredients:
- 1 cup dried chickpeas
- ½ onion, chopped
- 1 clove garlic
- ¼ cup fresh parsley leaves
- 1 teaspoon salt
- ¼ teaspoon crushed red pepper flakes
- 1 teaspoon ground cumin
- ½ teaspoon ground coriander
- 1 to 2 tablespoons flour
- olive oil
- Tomato Salad
- 2 tomatoes, seeds removed and diced
- ½ cucumber, finely diced
- ¼ red onion, finely diced and rinsed with water
- 1 teaspoon red wine vinegar
- 1 tablespoon olive oil
- salt and freshly ground black pepper
- 2 tablespoons chopped fresh parsley

Directions:
1. Cover the chickpeas with water and let them soak overnight on the counter. Then drain the chickpeas and put them in a food processor,

along with the onion, garlic, parsley, spices and 1 tablespoon of flour. Pulse in the food processor until the mixture has broken down into a coarse paste consistency. The mixture should hold together when you pinch it. Add more flour as needed, until you get this consistency.

2. Scoop portions of the mixture (about 2 tablespoons in size) and shape into balls. Place the balls on a plate and refrigerate for at least 30 minutes. You should have between 12 and 14 balls.

3. Preheat the air fryer to 380°F.

4. Spray the falafel balls with oil and place them in the air fryer. Air-fry for 10 minutes, rolling them over and spraying them with oil again halfway through the cooking time so that they cook and brown evenly.

5. Serve with pita bread, hummus, cucumbers, hot peppers, tomatoes or any other fillings you might like.

Bite-sized Blooming Onions

Servings: 4

Cooking Time: 35 Minutes + Cooling Time

Ingredients:
- 1 lb cipollini onions
- 1 cup flour
- 1 tsp salt
- ½ tsp paprika
- 1 tsp cayenne pepper
- 2 eggs
- 2 tbsp milk

Directions:

1. Preheat the air fryer to 375°F. Carefully peel the onions and cut a ½ inch off the stem ends and trim the root ends. Place them root-side down on the cutting surface and cut the onions into quarters. Be careful not to cut al the way to the bottom. Cut each quarter into 2 sections and pull the wedges apart without breaking them.

2. In a shallow bowl, add the flour, salt, paprika, and cayenne, and in a separate shallow bowl, beat the eggs with the milk. Dip the onions in the flour, then dip in the egg mix, coating evenly, and then in the flour mix again. Shake off excess flour. Put the onions in the frying basket, cut-side up, and spray with cooking oil. Air Fry for 10-15 minutes until the onions are crispy on

the outside, tender on the inside. Let cool for 10 minutes, then serve.

Meatless Kimchi Bowls

Servings: 4

Cooking Time: 20 Minutes

Ingredients:
- 2 cups canned chickpeas
- 1 carrot, julienned
- 6 scallions, sliced
- 1 zucchini, diced
- 2 tbsp coconut aminos
- 2 tsp sesame oil
- 1 tsp rice vinegar
- 2 tsp granulated sugar
- 1 tbsp gochujang
- ¼ tsp salt
- ½ cup kimchi
- 2 tsp roasted sesame seeds

Directions:

1. Preheat air fryer to 350ºF. Combine all ingredients, except for the kimchi, 2 scallions, and sesame seeds, in a baking pan. Place the pan in the frying basket and Air Fry for 6 minutes. Toss in kimchi and cook for 2 more minutes. Divide between 2 bowls and garnish with the remaining scallions and sesame seeds. Serve immediately.

Italian Stuffed Bell Peppers

Servings: 4

Cooking Time: 75 Minutes

Ingredients:
- 4 green and red bell peppers, tops and insides discarded
- 2 russet potatoes, scrubbed and perforated with a fork
- 2 tsp olive oil
- 2 Italian sausages, cubed
- 2 tbsp milk
- 2 tbsp yogurt
- 1 tsp olive oil
- 1 tbsp Italian seasoning
- Salt and pepper to taste
- ¼ cup canned corn kernels
- ½ cup mozzarella shreds
- 2 tsp chopped parsley
- 1 cup bechamel sauce

Directions:

1. Preheat air fryer at 400°F. Rub olive oil over both potatoes and sprinkle with salt and pepper. Place them in the frying basket and Bake for 45 minutes, flipping at 30 minutes mark. Let cool onto a cutting board for 5 minutes until cool enough to handle. Scoop out cooled potato into a bowl. Discard skins.

2. Place Italian sausages in the frying basket and Air Fry for 2 minutes. Using the back of a fork, mash cooked potatoes, yogurt, milk, olive oil, Italian seasoning, salt, and pepper until smooth. Toss in cooked sausages, corn, and mozzarella cheese. Stuff bell peppers with the potato mixture. Place bell peppers in the frying basket and Bake for 10 minutes. Serve immediately sprinkled with parsley and bechamel sauce on side.

Chicano Rice Bowls

Servings: 4
Cooking Time: 10 Minutes

Ingredients:
- 1 cup sour cream
- 2 tbsp milk
- 1 tsp ground cumin
- 1 tsp chili powder
- 1/8 tsp cayenne pepper
- 1 tbsp tomato paste
- 1 white onion, chopped
- 1 clove garlic, minced
- ½ tsp ground turmeric
- ½ tsp salt
- 1 cup canned black beans
- 1 cup canned corn kernels
- 1 tsp olive oil
- 4 cups cooked brown rice
- 3 tomatoes, diced
- 1 avocado, diced

Directions:

1. Whisk the sour cream, milk, cumin, ground turmeric, chili powder, cayenne pepper, and salt in a bowl. Let chill covered in the fridge until ready to use.

2. Preheat air fryer at 350°F. Combine beans, white onion, tomato paste, garlic, corn, and olive oil in a bowl. Transfer it into the frying basket and Air Fry for 5 minutes. Divide cooked rice into 4 serving bowls. Top each with bean mix-

ture, tomatoes, and avocado and drizzle with sour cream mixture over. Serve immediately.

Berbere Eggplant Dip

Servings: 4
Cooking Time: 35 Minutes

Ingredients:
- 1 eggplant, halved lengthwise
- 3 tsp olive oil
- 2 tsp pine nuts
- ¼ cup tahini
- 1 tbsp lemon juice
- 2 cloves garlic, minced
- ¼ tsp berbere seasoning
- ⅛ tsp ground cumin
- Salt and pepper to taste
- 1 tbsp chopped parsley

Directions:

1. Preheat air fryer to 370°F. Brush the eggplant with some olive oil. With a fork, pierce the eggplant flesh a few times. Place them, flat sides-down, in the frying basket. Air Fry for 25 minutes. Transfer the eggplant to a cutting board and let cool for 3 minutes until easy to handle. Place pine nuts in the frying basket and Air Fry for 2 minutes, shaking every 30 seconds. Set aside in a bowl.

2. Scoop out the eggplant flesh and add to a food processor. Add in tahini, lemon juice, garlic, berbere seasoning, cumin, salt, and black pepper and pulse until smooth. Transfer to a serving bowl. Scatter with toasted pine nuts, parsley, and the remaining olive oil. Serve immediately.

Cheddar-bean Flautas

Servings: 4
Cooking Time: 15 Minutes

Ingredients:
- 8 corn tortillas
- 1 can refried beans
- 1 cup shredded cheddar
- 1 cup guacamole

Directions:

1. Preheat air fryer to 390°F. Wet the tortillas with water. Spray the frying basket with oil and stack the tortillas inside. Air Fry for 1 minute.

Remove to a flat surface, laying them out individually. Scoop an equal amount of beans in a line down the center of each tortilla. Top with cheddar cheese. Roll the tortilla sides over the filling and put seam-side down in the greased frying basket. Air Fry for 7 minutes or until the tortillas are golden and crispy. Serve immediately topped with guacamole.

Golden Fried Tofu

Servings: 4
Cooking Time: 20 Minutes

Ingredients:
- ¼ cup flour
- ¼ cup cornstarch
- 1 tsp garlic powder
- ¼ tsp onion powder
- Salt and pepper to taste
- 1 firm tofu, cubed
- 2 tbsp cilantro, chopped

Directions:
1. Preheat air fryer to 390°F. Combine the flour, cornstarch, salt, garlic, onion powder, and black pepper in a bowl. Stir well. Place the tofu cubes in the flour mix. Toss to coat. Spray the tofu with oil and place them in a single layer in the greased frying basket. Air Fry for 14-16 minutes, flipping the pieces once until golden and crunchy. Top with freshly chopped cilantro and serve immediately.

Caprese-style Sandwiches

Servings: 2
Cooking Time: 20 Minutes

Ingredients:
- 2 tbsp balsamic vinegar
- 4 sandwich bread slices
- 2 oz mozzarella shreds
- 3 tbsp pesto sauce
- 2 tomatoes, sliced
- 8 basil leaves
- 8 baby spinach leaves
- 2 tbsp olive oil

Directions:
1. Preheat air fryer at 350°F. Drizzle balsamic vinegar on the bottom of bread slices and smear with pesto sauce. Then, layer mozzarella cheese, tomatoes, baby spinach leaves and basil leaves on top. Add top bread slices. Rub the outside top and bottom of each sandwich with olive oil. Place them in the frying basket and Bake for 5 minutes, flipping once. Serve right away.

Sesame Orange Tofu With Snow Peas

Servings: 4
Cooking Time: 40 Minutes

Ingredients:
- 14 oz tofu, cubed
- 1 tbsp tamari
- 1 tsp olive oil
- 1 tsp sesame oil
- 1 ½ tbsp cornstarch, divided
- ½ tsp salt
- ¼ tsp garlic powder
- 1 cup snow peas
- ½ cup orange juice
- ¼ cup vegetable broth
- 1 orange, zested
- 1 garlic clove, minced
- ¼ tsp ground ginger
- 2 scallions, chopped
- 1 tbsp sesame seeds
- 2 cups cooked jasmine rice
- 2 tbsp chopped parsley

Directions:
1. Preheat air fryer to 400°F. Combine tofu, tamari, olive oil, and sesame oil in a large bowl until tofu is coated. Add in 1 tablespoon cornstarch, salt, and garlic powder and toss. Arrange the tofu on the frying basket. Air Fry for 5 minutes, then shake the basket. Add snow peas and Air Fry for 5 minutes. Place tofu mixture in a bowl.
2. Bring the orange juice, vegetable broth, orange zest, garlic, and ginger to a boil over medium heat in a small saucepan. Whisk the rest of the cornstarch and 1 tablespoon water in a small bowl to make a slurry. Pour the slurry into the saucepan and constantly stir for 2 minutes until the sauce has thickened. Let off the heat for 2 minutes. Pour the orange sauce, scallions, and sesame seeds in the bowl with the tofu and stir to coat. Serve with jasmine rice sprinkled with parsley. Enjoy!

Golden Breaded Mushrooms

Servings: 2
Cooking Time: 20 Minutes

Ingredients:

- 2 cups crispy rice cereal
- 1 tsp nutritional yeast
- 2 tsp garlic powder
- 1tsp dried oregano
- 1 tsp dried basil
- Salt to taste
- 1 tbsp Dijon mustard
- 1 tbsp mayonnaise
- ¼ cup milk
- 8 oz whole mushrooms
- 4 tbsp chili sauce
- 3 tbsp mayonnaise

Directions:

1. Preheat air fryer at 350°F. Blend rice cereal, garlic powder, oregano, basil, nutritional yeast, and salt in a food processor until it gets a breadcrumb consistency. Set aside in a bowl. Mix the mustard, mayonnaise, and milk in a bowl. Dip mushrooms in the mustard mixture; shake off any excess. Then, dredge them in the breadcrumbs; shake off any excess. Places mushrooms in the greased frying basket and Air Fry for 7 minutes, shaking once. Mix the mayonnaise with chili sauce in a small bowl. Serve the mushrooms with the dipping sauce on the side.

Quinoa Burgers With Feta Cheese And Dill

Servings: 6
Cooking Time: 10 Minutes

Ingredients:

- 1 cup quinoa (red, white or multi-colored)
- 1½ cups water
- 1 teaspoon salt
- freshly ground black pepper
- 1½ cups rolled oats
- 3 eggs, lightly beaten
- ¼ cup minced white onion
- ½ cup crumbled feta cheese
- ¼ cup chopped fresh dill
- salt and freshly ground black pepper
- vegetable or canola oil, in a spray bottle
- whole-wheat hamburger buns (or gluten-free hamburger buns*)
- arugula
- tomato, sliced
- red onion, sliced
- mayonnaise

Directions:

1. Make the quinoa: Rinse the quinoa in cold water in a saucepan, swirling it with your hand until any dry husks rise to the surface. Drain the quinoa as well as you can and then put the saucepan on the stovetop to dry and toast the quinoa. Turn the heat to medium-high and shake the pan regularly until you see the quinoa moving easily and can hear the seeds moving in the pan, indicating that they are dry. Add the water, salt and pepper. Bring the liquid to a boil and then reduce the heat to low or medium-low. You should see just a few bubbles, not a boil. Cover with a lid, leaving it askew and simmer for 20 minutes. Turn the heat off and fluff the quinoa with a fork. If there's any liquid left in the bottom of the pot, place it back on the burner for another 3 minutes or so. Spread the cooked quinoa out on a sheet pan to cool.

2. Combine the room temperature quinoa in a large bowl with the oats, eggs, onion, cheese and dill. Season with salt and pepper and mix well (remember that feta cheese is salty). Shape the mixture into 6 patties with flat sides (so they fit more easily into the air fryer). Add a little water or a few more rolled oats if necessary to get the mixture to be the right consistency to make patties.

3. Preheat the air-fryer to 400°F.

4. Spray both sides of the patties generously with oil and transfer them to the air fryer basket in one layer (you will probably have to cook these burgers in batches, depending on the size of your air fryer). Air-fry each batch at 400°F for 10 minutes, flipping the burgers over halfway through the cooking time.

5. Build your burger on the whole-wheat hamburger buns with arugula, tomato, red onion and mayonnaise.

Vegan French Toast

Servings: 4
Cooking Time: 15 Minutes

Ingredients:
- 1 ripe banana, mashed
- ¼ cup protein powder
- ½ cup milk
- 2 tbsp ground flaxseed
- 4 bread slices
- 2 tbsp agave syrup

Directions:
1. Preheat air fryer to 370°F. Combine the banana, protein powder, milk, and flaxseed in a shallow bowl and mix well Dip bread slices into the mixture. Place the slices on a lightly greased pan in a single layer and pour any of the remaining mixture evenly over the bread. Air Fry for 10 minutes, or until golden brown and crispy, flipping once. Serve warm topped with agave syrup.

Cheddar Bean Taquitos

Servings: 4
Cooking Time: 25 Minutes

Ingredients:
- 1 cup refried beans
- 2 cups cheddar shreds
- ½ jalapeño pepper, minced
- ¼ chopped white onion
- 1 tsp oregano
- 15 soft corn tortillas

Directions:
1. Preheat air fryer at 350°F. Spread refried beans, jalapeño pepper, white onion, oregano and cheddar shreds down the center of each corn tortilla. Roll each tortilla tightly. Place tacos, seam side down, in the frying basket, and Air Fry for 4 minutes. Serve immediately.

Pizza Portobello Mushrooms

Servings: 2
Cooking Time: 18 Minutes

Ingredients:
- 2 portobello mushroom caps, gills removed (see Figure 13-1)
- 1 teaspoon extra-virgin olive oil
- ¼ cup diced onion
- 1 teaspoon minced garlic
- 1 medium zucchini, shredded
- 1 teaspoon dried oregano
- ½ teaspoon black pepper
- ¼ teaspoon salt
- ⅓ cup marinara sauce
- ¼ cup shredded part-skim mozzarella cheese
- ¼ teaspoon red pepper flakes
- 2 tablespoons Parmesan cheese
- 2 tablespoons chopped basil

Directions:
1. Preheat the air fryer to 370°F.
2. Lightly spray the mushrooms with an olive oil mist and place into the air fryer to cook for 10 minutes, cap side up.
3. Add the olive oil to a pan and sauté the onion and garlic together for about 2 to 4 minutes. Stir in the zucchini, oregano, pepper, and salt, and continue to cook. When the zucchini has cooked down (usually about 4 to 6 minutes), add in the marinara sauce. Remove from the heat and stir in the mozzarella cheese.
4. Remove the mushrooms from the air fryer basket when cooking completes. Reset the temperature to 350°F.
5. Using a spoon, carefully stuff the mushrooms with the zucchini marinara mixture.
6. Return the stuffed mushrooms to the air fryer basket and cook for 5 to 8 minutes, or until the cheese is lightly browned. You should be able to easily insert a fork into the mushrooms when they're cooked.
7. Remove the mushrooms and sprinkle the red pepper flakes, Parmesan cheese, and fresh basil over the top.
8. Serve warm.

Green Bean & Baby Potato Mix

Servings: 4
Cooking Time: 25 Minutes

Ingredients:
- 1 lb baby potatoes, halved
- 4 garlic cloves, minced
- 2 tbsp olive oil
- Salt and pepper to taste
- ½ tsp hot paprika
- ½ tbsp taco seasoning
- 1 tbsp chopped parsley
- ½ lb green beans, trimmed

Directions:
1. Preheat air fryer to 375°F. Toss potatoes, garlic, olive oil, salt, pepper, hot paprika, and taco seasoning in a large bowl. Arrange the potatoes in a single layer in the air fryer basket. Air Fry for 10 minutes, then stir in green beans. Air Fry for another 10 minutes. Serve hot sprinkled with parsley.

Asparagus, Mushroom And Cheese Soufflés

Servings: 3
Cooking Time: 21 Minutes

Ingredients:
- butter
- grated Parmesan cheese
- 3 button mushrooms, thinly sliced
- 8 spears asparagus, sliced ½-inch long
- 1 teaspoon olive oil
- 1 tablespoon butter
- 4½ teaspoons flour
- pinch paprika
- pinch ground nutmeg
- salt and freshly ground black pepper
- ½ cup milk
- ½ cup grated Gruyère cheese or other Swiss cheese (about 2 ounces)
- 2 eggs, separated

Directions:
1. Butter three 6-ounce ramekins and dust with grated Parmesan cheese. (Butter the ramekins and then coat the butter with Parmesan by shaking it around in the ramekin and dumping out any excess.)

2. Preheat the air fryer to 400°F.
3. Toss the mushrooms and asparagus in a bowl with the olive oil. Transfer the vegetables to the air fryer and air-fry for 7 minutes, shaking the basket once or twice to redistribute the Ingredients while they cook.
4. While the vegetables are cooking, make the soufflé base. Melt the butter in a saucepan on the stovetop over medium heat. Add the flour, stir and cook for a minute or two. Add the paprika, nutmeg, salt and pepper. Whisk in the milk and bring the mixture to a simmer to thicken. Remove the pan from the heat and add the cheese, stirring to melt. Let the mixture cool for just a few minutes and then whisk the egg yolks in, one at a time. Stir in the cooked mushrooms and asparagus. Let this soufflé base cool.
5. In a separate bowl, whisk the egg whites to soft peak stage (the point at which the whites can almost stand up on the end of your whisk). Fold the whipped egg whites into the soufflé base, adding a little at a time.
6. Preheat the air fryer to 330°F.
7. Transfer the batter carefully to the buttered ramekins, leaving about ½-inch at the top. Place the ramekins into the air fryer basket and air-fry for 14 minutes. The soufflés should have risen nicely and be brown on top. Serve immediately.

Vegetarian Shepherd´s Pie

Servings: 4
Cooking Time: 40 Minutes

Ingredients:
- 1 russet potato, peeled and diced
- 1 tbsp olive oil
- 2 tbsp balsamic vinegar
- ¼ cup cheddar shreds
- 2 tbsp milk
- Salt and pepper to taste
- 2 tsp avocado oil
- 1 cup beefless grounds
- ½ onion, diced
- 3 cloves garlic
- 1 carrot, diced
- ¼ diced green bell peppers
- 1 celery stalk, diced
- 2/3 cup tomato sauce
- 1 tsp chopped rosemary
- 1 tbsp sesame seeds

- 1 tsp thyme leaves
- 1 lemon

Directions:

1. Add salted water to a pot over high heat and bring it to a boil. Add in diced potatoes and cook for 5 minutes until fork tender. Drain and transfer it to a bowl. Add in the olive oil cheddar shreds, milk, salt, and pepper and mash it until smooth. Set the potato topping aside.

2. Preheat air fryer at 350°F. Place avocado oil, beefless grounds, garlic, onion, carrot, bell pepper, and celery in a skillet over medium heat and cook for 4 minutes until the veggies are tender. Stir in the remaining ingredients and turn the heat off. Spoon the filling into a greased cake pan. Top with the potato topping.

3. Using tines of a fork, create shallow lines along the top of mashed potatoes. Place cake pan in the frying basket and Bake for 12 minutes. Let rest for 10 minutes before serving sprinkled with sesame seeds and squeezed lemon.

Fried Rice With Curried Tofu

Servings: 4
Cooking Time: 25 Minutes

Ingredients:

- 8 oz extra-firm tofu, cubed
- ½ cup canned coconut milk
- 2 tsp red curry paste
- 2 cloves garlic, minced
- 1 tbsp avocado oil
- 1 tbsp coconut oil
- 2 cups cooked rice
- 1 tbsp turmeric powder
- Salt and pepper to taste
- 4 lime wedges
- ¼ cup chopped cilantro

Directions:

1. Preheat air fryer to 350°F. Combine tofu, coconut milk, curry paste, garlic, and avocado oil in a bowl. Pour the mixture into a baking pan. Place the pan in the frying basket and Air Fry for 10 minutes, stirring once.

2. Melt the coconut oil in a skillet over medium heat. Add in rice, turmeric powder, salt, and black pepper, and cook for 2 minutes or until heated through. Divide the cooked rice between 4 medium bowls and top with tofu mixture and sauce. Top with cilantro and lime wedges to serve.

Sweet Roasted Carrots

Servings: 4
Cooking Time: 25 Minutes

Ingredients:

- 6 carrots, cut into ½-inch pieces
- 2 tbsp butter, melted
- 2 tbsp parsley, chopped
- 1 tsp honey

Directions:

1. Preheat air fryer to 390°F. Add carrots to a baking pan and pour over butter, honey, and 2-3 tbsp of water. Mix well. Transfer the carrots to the greased frying basket and Roast for 12 minutes, shaking the basket once. Sprinkle with parsley and serve warm.

Vegetarian Stuffed Bell Peppers

Servings: 3
Cooking Time: 40 Minutes

Ingredients:

- 1 cup mushrooms, chopped
- 1 tbsp allspice
- ¾ cup Alfredo sauce
- ½ cup canned diced tomatoes
- 1 cup cooked rice
- 2 tbsp dried parsley
- 2 tbsp hot sauce
- Salt and pepper to taste
- 3 large bell peppers

Directions:

1. Preheat air fryer to 375°F. Whisk mushrooms, allspice and 1 cup of boiling water until smooth. Stir in Alfredo sauce, tomatoes and juices, rice, parsley, hot sauce, salt, and black pepper. Set aside. Cut the top of each bell pepper, take out the core and seeds without breaking the pepper. Fill each pepper with the rice mixture and cover them with a 6-inch square of aluminum foil, folding the edges. Roast for 30 minutes until tender. Let cool completely before unwrapping. Serve immediately.

Lentil Fritters

Servings: 9
Cooking Time: 12 Minutes

Ingredients:
- 1 cup cooked red lentils
- 1 cup riced cauliflower
- ½ medium zucchini, shredded (about 1 cup)
- ¼ cup finely chopped onion
- ¼ teaspoon salt
- ¼ teaspoon black pepper
- ½ teaspoon garlic powder
- ¼ teaspoon paprika
- 1 large egg
- ⅓ cup quinoa flour

Directions:
1. Preheat the air fryer to 370°F.
2. In a large bowl, mix the lentils, cauliflower, zucchini, onion, salt, pepper, garlic powder, and paprika. Mix in the egg and flour until a thick dough forms.
3. Using a large spoon, form the dough into 9 large fritters.
4. Liberally spray the air fryer basket with olive oil. Place the fritters into the basket, leaving space around each fritter so you can flip them.
5. Cook for 6 minutes, flip, and cook another 6 minutes.
6. Remove from the air fryer and repeat with the remaining fritters. Serve warm with desired sauce and sides.

Pine Nut Eggplant Dip

Servings: 4
Cooking Time: 35 Minutes

Ingredients:
- 2 ½ tsp olive oil
- 1 eggplant, halved lengthwise
- 1/2 cup Parmesan cheese
- 2 tsp pine nuts
- 1 tbsp chopped walnuts
- ¼ cup tahini
- 1 tbsp lemon juice
- 2 cloves garlic, minced
- 1/8 tsp ground cumin
- 1 tsp smoked paprika
- Salt and pepper to taste
- 1 tbsp chopped parsley

Directions:
1. Preheat air fryer at 375°F. Rub olive oil over eggplant and pierce the eggplant flesh 3 times with a fork. Place eggplant, flat side down, in the frying basket and Bake for 25 minutes. Let cool onto a cutting board for 5 minutes until cool enough to handle. Scoop out eggplant flesh. Add pine nuts and walnuts to the basket and Air Fry for 2 minutes, shaking every 30 seconds to ensure they don't burn. Set aside in a bowl.
2. In a food processor, blend eggplant flesh, tahini, lemon juice, garlic, smoked paprika, cumin, salt, and pepper until smooth. Transfer to a bowl. Scatter with the roasted pine nuts, Parmesan cheese, and parsley. Drizzle the dip with the remaining olive oil. Serve and enjoy!

Sandwiches And Burgers Recipes

Best-ever Roast Beef Sandwiches 72
Asian Glazed Meatballs 72
Black Bean Veggie Burgers 73
Thai-style Pork Sliders 73
Thanksgiving Turkey Sandwiches...............................74
Lamb Burgers 74
Chicken Club Sandwiches 75
Inside-out Cheeseburgers...............................75
Provolone Stuffed Meatballs 76
Chicken Gyros 76
Philly Cheesesteak Sandwiches 77
Inside Out Cheeseburgers 77
Mexican Cheeseburgers 77
Salmon Burgers 78
Crunchy Falafel Balls 78
Chicken Saltimbocca Sandwiches 79
White Bean Veggie Burgers...............................79
Chicken Apple Brie Melt...............................80
Chicken Spiedies 80
Perfect Burgers 81
Sausage And Pepper Heros 81
Eggplant Parmesan Subs 82
Dijon Thyme Burgers 82
Reuben Sandwiches 83
Chili Cheese Dogs 83

Best-ever Roast Beef Sandwiches

Servings: 6
Cooking Time: 30-50 Minutes

Ingredients:
- 2½ teaspoons Olive oil
- 1½ teaspoons Dried oregano
- 1½ teaspoons Dried thyme
- 1½ teaspoons Onion powder
- 1½ teaspoons Table salt
- 1½ teaspoons Ground black pepper
- 3 pounds Beef eye of round
- 6 Round soft rolls, such as Kaiser rolls or hamburger buns (gluten-free, if a concern), split open lengthwise
- ¾ cup Regular, low-fat, or fat-free mayonnaise (gluten-free, if a concern)
- 6 Romaine lettuce leaves, rinsed
- 6 Round tomato slices (¼ inch thick)

Directions:
1. Preheat the air fryer to 350°F .
2. Mix the oil, oregano, thyme, onion powder, salt, and pepper in a small bowl. Spread this mixture all over the eye of round.
3. When the machine is at temperature, set the beef in the basket and air-fry for 30 to 50 minutes (the range depends on the size of the cut), turning the meat twice, until an instant-read meat thermometer inserted into the thickest piece of the meat registers 130°F for rare, 140°F for medium, or 150°F for well-done.
4. Use kitchen tongs to transfer the beef to a cutting board. Cool for 10 minutes. If serving now, carve into ⅛-inch-thick slices. Spread each roll with 2 tablespoons mayonnaise and divide the beef slices between the rolls. Top with a lettuce leaf and a tomato slice and serve. Or set the beef in a container, cover, and refrigerate for up to 3 days to make cold roast beef sandwiches anytime.

Asian Glazed Meatballs

Servings: 4
Cooking Time: 10 Minutes

Ingredients:
- 1 large shallot, finely chopped
- 2 cloves garlic, minced
- 1 tablespoon grated fresh ginger
- 2 teaspoons fresh thyme, finely chopped
- 1½ cups brown mushrooms, very finely chopped (a food processor works well here)
- 2 tablespoons soy sauce
- freshly ground black pepper
- 1 pound ground beef
- ½ pound ground pork
- 3 egg yolks
- 1 cup Thai sweet chili sauce (spring roll sauce)
- ¼ cup toasted sesame seeds
- 2 scallions, sliced

Directions:
1. Combine the shallot, garlic, ginger, thyme, mushrooms, soy sauce, freshly ground black pepper, ground beef and pork, and egg yolks in a bowl and mix the ingredients together. Gently shape the mixture into 24 balls, about the size of a golf ball.
2. Preheat the air fryer to 380°F.
3. Working in batches, air-fry the meatballs for 8 minutes, turning the meatballs over halfway through the cooking time. Drizzle some of the Thai sweet chili sauce on top of each meatball and return the basket to the air fryer, air-frying for another 2 minutes. Reserve the remaining Thai sweet chili sauce for serving.
4. As soon as the meatballs are done, sprinkle with toasted sesame seeds and transfer them to a serving platter. Scatter the scallions around and serve warm.

Black Bean Veggie Burgers

Servings: 3
Cooking Time: 10 Minutes

Ingredients:
- 1 cup Drained and rinsed canned black beans
- ⅓ cup Pecan pieces
- ⅓ cup Rolled oats (not quick-cooking or steel-cut; gluten-free, if a concern)
- 2 tablespoons (or 1 small egg) Pasteurized egg substitute, such as Egg Beaters (gluten-free, if a concern)
- 2 teaspoons Red ketchup-like chili sauce, such as Heinz
- ¼ teaspoon Ground cumin
- ¼ teaspoon Dried oregano
- ¼ teaspoon Table salt
- ¼ teaspoon Ground black pepper
- Olive oil
- Olive oil spray

Directions:
1. Preheat the air fryer to 400°F.
2. Put the beans, pecans, oats, egg substitute or egg, chili sauce, cumin, oregano, salt, and pepper in a food processor. Cover and process to a coarse paste that will hold its shape like sugar-cookie dough, adding olive oil in 1-teaspoon increments to get the mixture to blend smoothly. The amount of olive oil is actually dependent on the internal moisture content of the beans and the oats. Figure on about 1 tablespoon (three 1-teaspoon additions) for the smaller batch, with proportional increases for the other batches. A little too much olive oil can't hurt, but a dry paste will fall apart as it cooks and a far-too-wet paste will stick to the basket.
3. Scrape down and remove the blade. Using clean, wet hands, form the paste into two 4-inch patties for the small batch, three 4-inch patties for the medium, or four 4-inch patties for the large batch, setting them one by one on a cutting board. Generously coat both sides of the patties with olive oil spray.
4. Set them in the basket in one layer. Air-fry undisturbed for 10 minutes, or until lightly browned and crisp at the edges.
5. Use a nonstick-safe spatula, and perhaps a flatware fork for balance, to transfer the burgers to a wire rack. Cool for 5 minutes before serving.

Thai-style Pork Sliders

Servings: 4
Cooking Time: 15 Minutes

Ingredients:
- 11 ounces Ground pork
- 2½ tablespoons Very thinly sliced scallions, white and green parts
- 4 teaspoons Minced peeled fresh ginger
- 2½ teaspoons Fish sauce (gluten-free, if a concern)
- 2 teaspoons Thai curry paste (see the head-note; gluten-free, if a concern)
- 2 teaspoons Light brown sugar
- ¾ teaspoon Ground black pepper
- 4 Slider buns (gluten-free, if a concern)

Directions:
1. Preheat the air fryer to 375°F.
2. Gently mix the pork, scallions, ginger, fish sauce, curry paste, brown sugar, and black pepper in a bowl until well combined. With clean, wet hands, form about ⅓ cup of the pork mixture into a slider about 2½ inches in diameter. Repeat until you use up all the meat—3 sliders for the small batch, 4 for the medium, and 6 for the large. (Keep wetting your hands to help the patties adhere.)
3. When the machine is at temperature, set the sliders in the basket in one layer. Air-fry undisturbed for 14 minutes, or until the sliders are golden brown and caramelized at their edges and an instant-read meat thermometer inserted into the center of a slider registers 160°F.
4. Use a nonstick-safe spatula, and perhaps a flatware fork for balance, to transfer the sliders to a cutting board. Set the buns cut side down in the basket in one layer (working in batches as necessary) and air-fry undisturbed for 1 minute, to toast a bit and warm up. Serve the sliders warm in the buns.

Thanksgiving Turkey Sandwiches

Servings: 3

Cooking Time: 10 Minutes

Ingredients:
- 1½ cups Herb-seasoned stuffing mix (not corn-bread-style; gluten-free, if a concern)
- 1 Large egg white(s)
- 2 tablespoons Water
- 3 5- to 6-ounce turkey breast cutlets
- Vegetable oil spray
- 4½ tablespoons Purchased cranberry sauce, preferably whole berry
- ⅛ teaspoon Ground cinnamon
- ⅛ teaspoon Ground dried ginger
- 4½ tablespoons Regular, low-fat, or fat-free mayonnaise (gluten-free, if a concern)
- 6 tablespoons Shredded Brussels sprouts
- 3 Kaiser rolls (gluten-free, if a concern), split open

Directions:
1. Preheat the air fryer to 375°F.
2. Put the stuffing mix in a heavy zip-closed bag, seal it, lay it flat on your counter, and roll a rolling pin over the bag to crush the stuffing mix to the consistency of rough sand. (Or you can pulse the stuffing mix to the desired consistency in a food processor.)
3. Set up and fill two shallow soup plates or small pie plates on your counter: one for the egg white(s), whisked with the water until foamy; and one for the ground stuffing mix.
4. Dip a cutlet in the egg white mixture, coating both sides and letting any excess egg white slip back into the rest. Set the cutlet in the ground stuffing mix and coat it evenly on both sides, pressing gently to coat well on both sides. Lightly coat the cutlet on both sides with vegetable oil spray, set it aside, and continue dipping and coating the remaining cutlets in the same way.
5. Set the cutlets in the basket and air-fry undisturbed for 10 minutes, or until crisp and brown. Use kitchen tongs to transfer the cutlets to a wire rack to cool for a few minutes.
6. Meanwhile, stir the cranberry sauce with the cinnamon and ginger in a small bowl. Mix the shredded Brussels sprouts and mayonnaise in a second bowl until the vegetable is evenly coated.

7. Build the sandwiches by spreading about 1½ tablespoons of the cranberry mixture on the cut side of the bottom half of each roll. Set a cutlet on top, then spread about 3 tablespoons of the Brussels sprouts mixture evenly over the cutlet. Set the other half of the roll on top and serve warm.

Lamb Burgers

Servings: 3

Cooking Time: 17 Minutes

Ingredients:
- 1 pound 2 ounces Ground lamb
- 3 tablespoons Crumbled feta
- 1 teaspoon Minced garlic
- 1 teaspoon Tomato paste
- ¾ teaspoon Ground coriander
- ¾ teaspoon Ground dried ginger
- Up to ⅛ teaspoon Cayenne
- Up to a ⅛ teaspoon Table salt (optional)
- 3 Kaiser rolls or hamburger buns (gluten-free, if a concern), split open

Directions:
1. Preheat the air fryer to 375°F.
2. Gently mix the ground lamb, feta, garlic, tomato paste, coriander, ginger, cayenne, and salt (if using) in a bowl until well combined, trying to keep the bits of cheese intact. Form this mixture into two 5-inch patties for the small batch, three 5-inch patties for the medium, or four 5-inch patties for the large.
3. Set the patties in the basket in one layer and air-fry undisturbed for 16 minutes, or until an instant-read meat thermometer inserted into one burger registers 160°F. (The cheese is not an issue with the temperature probe in this recipe as it was for the Inside-Out Cheeseburgers, because the feta is so well mixed into the ground meat.)
4. Use a nonstick-safe spatula, and perhaps a flatware fork for balance, to transfer the burgers to a cutting board. Set the buns cut side down in the basket in one layer (working in batches as necessary) and air-fry undisturbed for 1 minute, to toast a bit and warm up. Serve the burgers warm in the buns.

Chicken Club Sandwiches

Servings: 3
Cooking Time: 15 Minutes

Ingredients:
- 3 5- to 6-ounce boneless skinless chicken breasts
- 6 Thick-cut bacon strips (gluten-free, if a concern)
- 3 Long soft rolls, such as hero, hoagie, or Italian sub rolls (gluten-free, if a concern)
- 3 tablespoons Regular, low-fat, or fat-free mayonnaise (gluten-free, if a concern)
- 3 Lettuce leaves, preferably romaine or iceberg
- 6 ¼-inch-thick tomato slices

Directions:
1. Preheat the air fryer to 375°F.
2. Wrap each chicken breast with 2 strips of bacon, spiraling the bacon around the meat, slightly overlapping the strips on each revolution. Start the second strip of bacon farther down the breast but on a line with the start of the first strip so they both end at a lined-up point on the chicken breast.
3. When the machine is at temperature, set the wrapped breasts bacon-seam side down in the basket with space between them. Air-fry undisturbed for 12 minutes, until the bacon is browned, crisp, and cooked through and an instant-read meat thermometer inserted into the center of a breast registers 165°F. You may need to add 2 minutes in the air fryer if the temperature is at 360°F.
4. Use kitchen tongs to transfer the breasts to a wire rack. Split the rolls open lengthwise and set them cut side down in the basket. Air-fry for 1 minute, or until warmed through.
5. Use kitchen tongs to transfer the rolls to a cutting board. Spread 1 tablespoon mayonnaise on the cut side of one half of each roll. Top with a chicken breast, lettuce leaf, and tomato slice. Serve warm.

Inside-out Cheeseburgers

Servings: 3
Cooking Time: 9-11 Minutes

Ingredients:
- 1 pound 2 ounces 90% lean ground beef
- ¾ teaspoon Dried oregano
- ¾ teaspoon Table salt
- ¾ teaspoon Ground black pepper
- ¼ teaspoon Garlic powder
- 6 tablespoons (about 1½ ounces) Shredded Cheddar, Swiss, or other semi-firm cheese, or a purchased blend of shredded cheeses
- 3 Hamburger buns (gluten-free, if a concern), split open

Directions:
1. Preheat the air fryer to 375°F.
2. Gently mix the ground beef, oregano, salt, pepper, and garlic powder in a bowl until well combined without turning the mixture to mush. Form it into two 6-inch patties for the small batch, three for the medium, or four for the large.
3. Place 2 tablespoons of the shredded cheese in the center of each patty. With clean hands, fold the sides of the patty up to cover the cheese, then pick it up and roll it gently into a ball to seal the cheese inside. Gently press it back into a 5-inch burger without letting any cheese squish out. Continue filling and preparing more burgers, as needed.
4. Place the burgers in the basket in one layer and air-fry undisturbed for 8 minutes for medium or 10 minutes for well-done. (An instant-read meat thermometer won't work for these burgers because it will hit the mostly melted cheese inside and offer a hotter temperature than the surrounding meat.)
5. Use a nonstick-safe spatula, and perhaps a flatware fork for balance, to transfer the burgers to a cutting board. Set the buns cut side down in the basket in one layer (working in batches as necessary) and air-fry undisturbed for 1 minute, to toast a bit and warm up. Cool the burgers a few minutes more, then serve them warm in the buns.

Provolone Stuffed Meatballs

Servings: 4
Cooking Time: 12 Minutes

Ingredients:
- 1 tablespoon olive oil
- 1 small onion, very finely chopped
- 1 to 2 cloves garlic, minced
- ¾ pound ground beef
- ¾ pound ground pork
- ¾ cup breadcrumbs
- ¼ cup grated Parmesan cheese
- ¼ cup finely chopped fresh parsley (or 1 tablespoon dried parsley)
- ½ teaspoon dried oregano
- 1½ teaspoons salt
- freshly ground black pepper
- 2 eggs, lightly beaten
- 5 ounces sharp or aged provolone cheese, cut into 1-inch cubes

Directions:
1. Preheat a skillet over medium-high heat. Add the oil and cook the onion and garlic until tender, but not browned.
2. Transfer the onion and garlic to a large bowl and add the beef, pork, breadcrumbs, Parmesan cheese, parsley, oregano, salt, pepper and eggs. Mix well until all the ingredients are combined. Divide the mixture into 12 evenly sized balls. Make one meatball at a time, by pressing a hole in the meatball mixture with your finger and pushing a piece of provolone cheese into the hole. Mold the meat back into a ball, enclosing the cheese.
3. Preheat the air fryer to 380°F.
4. Working in two batches, transfer six of the meatballs to the air fryer basket and air-fry for 12 minutes, shaking the basket and turning the meatballs a couple of times during the cooking process. Repeat with the remaining six meatballs. You can pop the first batch of meatballs into the air fryer for the last two minutes of cooking to re-heat them. Serve warm.

Chicken Gyros

Servings: 4
Cooking Time: 14 Minutes

Ingredients:
- 4 4- to 5-ounce boneless skinless chicken thighs, trimmed of any fat blobs
- 2 tablespoons Lemon juice
- 2 tablespoons Red wine vinegar
- 2 tablespoons Olive oil
- 2 teaspoons Dried oregano
- 2 teaspoons Minced garlic
- 1 teaspoon Table salt
- 1 teaspoon Ground black pepper
- 4 Pita pockets (gluten-free, if a concern)
- ½ cup Chopped tomatoes
- ½ cup Bottled regular, low-fat, or fat-free ranch dressing (gluten-free, if a concern)

Directions:
1. Mix the thighs, lemon juice, vinegar, oil, oregano, garlic, salt, and pepper in a zip-closed bag. Seal, gently massage the marinade into the meat through the plastic, and refrigerate for at least 2 hours or up to 6 hours. (Longer than that and the meat can turn rubbery.)
2. Set the plastic bag out on the counter (to make the contents a little less frigid). Preheat the air fryer to 375°F.
3. When the machine is at temperature, use kitchen tongs to place the thighs in the basket in one layer. Discard the marinade. Air-fry the chicken thighs undisturbed for 12 minutes, or until browned and an instant-read meat thermometer inserted into the thickest part of one thigh registers 165°F. You may need to air-fry the chicken 2 minutes longer if the machine's temperature is 360°F.
4. Use kitchen tongs to transfer the thighs to a cutting board. Cool for 5 minutes, then set one thigh in each of the pita pockets. Top each with 2 tablespoons chopped tomatoes and 2 tablespoons dressing. Serve warm.

Philly Cheesesteak Sandwiches

Servings: 3
Cooking Time: 9 Minutes

Ingredients:
- ¾ pound Shaved beef
- 1 tablespoon Worcestershire sauce (gluten-free, if a concern)
- ¼ teaspoon Garlic powder
- ¼ teaspoon Mild paprika
- 6 tablespoons (1½ ounces) Frozen bell pepper strips (do not thaw)
- 2 slices, broken into rings Very thin yellow or white medium onion slice(s)
- 6 ounces (6 to 8 slices) Provolone cheese slices
- 3 Long soft rolls such as hero, hoagie, or Italian sub rolls, or hot dog buns (gluten-free, if a concern), split open lengthwise

Directions:
1. Preheat the air fryer to 400°F.
2. When the machine is at temperature, spread the shaved beef in the basket, leaving a ½-inch perimeter around the meat for good air flow. Sprinkle the meat with the Worcestershire sauce, paprika, and garlic powder. Spread the peppers and onions on top of the meat.
3. Air-fry undisturbed for 6 minutes, or until cooked through. Set the cheese on top of the meat. Continue air-frying undisturbed for 3 minutes, or until the cheese has melted.
4. Use kitchen tongs to divide the meat and cheese layers in the basket between the rolls or buns. Serve hot.

Inside Out Cheeseburgers

Servings: 2
Cooking Time: 20 Minutes

Ingredients:
- ¾ pound lean ground beef
- 3 tablespoons minced onion
- 4 teaspoons ketchup
- 2 teaspoons yellow mustard
- salt and freshly ground black pepper
- 4 slices of Cheddar cheese, broken into smaller pieces
- 8 hamburger dill pickle chips

Directions:
1. Combine the ground beef, minced onion, ketchup, mustard, salt and pepper in a large bowl. Mix well to thoroughly combine the ingredients. Divide the meat into four equal portions.
2. To make the stuffed burgers, flatten each portion of meat into a thin patty. Place 4 pickle chips and half of the cheese onto the center of two of the patties, leaving a rim around the edge of the patty exposed. Place the remaining two patties on top of the first and press the meat together firmly, sealing the edges tightly. With the burgers on a flat surface, press the sides of the burger with the palm of your hand to create a straight edge. This will help keep the stuffing inside the burger while it cooks.
3. Preheat the air fryer to 370°F.
4. Place the burgers inside the air fryer basket and air-fry for 20 minutes, flipping the burgers over halfway through the cooking time.
5. Serve the cheeseburgers on buns with lettuce and tomato.

Mexican Cheeseburgers

Servings: 4
Cooking Time: 22 Minutes

Ingredients:
- 1¼ pounds ground beef
- ¼ cup finely chopped onion
- ½ cup crushed yellow corn tortilla chips
- 1 (1.25-ounce) packet taco seasoning
- ¼ cup canned diced green chilies
- 1 egg, lightly beaten
- 4 ounces pepper jack cheese, grated
- 4 (12-inch) flour tortillas
- shredded lettuce, sour cream, guacamole, salsa (for topping)

Directions:
1. Combine the ground beef, minced onion, crushed tortilla chips, taco seasoning, green chilies, and egg in a large bowl. Mix thoroughly until combined – your hands are good tools for this. Divide the meat into four equal portions and shape each portion into an oval-shaped burger.
2. Preheat the air fryer to 370°F.
3. Air-fry the burgers for 18 minutes, turning them over halfway through the cooking time. Divide the cheese between the burgers, lower fryer to 340°F and air-fry for an additional 4

minutes to melt the cheese. (This will give you a burger that is medium-well. If you prefer your cheeseburger medium-rare, shorten the cooking time to about 15 minutes and then add the cheese and proceed with the recipe.)

4. While the burgers are cooking, warm the tortillas wrapped in aluminum foil in a 350°F oven, or in a skillet with a little oil over medium-high heat for a couple of minutes. Keep the tortillas warm until the burgers are ready.

5. To assemble the burgers, spread sour cream over three quarters of the tortillas and top each with some shredded lettuce and salsa. Place the Mexican cheeseburgers on the lettuce and top with guacamole. Fold the tortillas around the burger, starting with the bottom and then folding the sides in over the top. (A little sour cream can help hold the seam of the tortilla together.) Serve immediately.

Salmon Burgers

Servings: 3
Cooking Time: 8 Minutes

Ingredients:
- 1 pound 2 ounces Skinless salmon fillet, preferably fattier Atlantic salmon
- 1½ tablespoons Minced chives or the green part of a scallion
- ½ cup Plain panko bread crumbs (gluten-free, if a concern)
- 1½ teaspoons Dijon mustard (gluten-free, if a concern)
- 1½ teaspoons Drained and rinsed capers, minced
- 1½ teaspoons Lemon juice
- ¼ teaspoon Table salt
- ¼ teaspoon Ground black pepper
- Vegetable oil spray

Directions:
1. Preheat the air fryer to 375°F .
2. Cut the salmon into pieces that will fit in a food processor. Cover and pulse until coarsely chopped. Add the chives and pulse to combine, until the fish is ground but not a paste. Scrape down and remove the blade. Scrape the salmon mixture into a bowl. Add the bread crumbs, mustard, capers, lemon juice, salt, and pepper. Stir gently until well combined.

3. Use clean and dry hands to form the mixture into two 5-inch patties for a small batch, three 5-inch patties for a medium batch, or four 5-inch patties for a large one.

4. Coat both sides of each patty with vegetable oil spray. Set them in the basket in one layer and air-fry undisturbed for 8 minutes, or until browned and an instant-read meat thermometer inserted into the center of a burger registers 145°F.

5. Use a nonstick-safe spatula, and perhaps a flatware fork for balance, to transfer the burgers to a wire rack. Cool for 2 or 3 minutes before serving.

Crunchy Falafel Balls

Servings: 8
Cooking Time: 16 Minutes

Ingredients:
- 2½ cups Drained and rinsed canned chickpeas
- ¼ cup Olive oil
- 3 tablespoons All-purpose flour
- 1½ teaspoons Dried oregano
- 1½ teaspoons Dried sage leaves
- 1½ teaspoons Dried thyme
- ¾ teaspoon Table salt
- Olive oil spray

Directions:
1. Preheat the air fryer to 400°F.
2. Place the chickpeas, olive oil, flour, oregano, sage, thyme, and salt in a food processor. Cover and process into a paste, stopping the machine at least once to scrape down the inside of the canister.
3. Scrape down and remove the blade. Using clean, wet hands, form 2 tablespoons of the paste into a ball, then continue making 9 more balls for a small batch, 15 more for a medium one, and 19 more for a large batch. Generously coat the balls in olive oil spray.
4. Set the balls in the basket in one layer with a little space between them and air-fry undisturbed for 16 minutes, or until well browned and crisp.
5. Dump the contents of the basket onto a wire rack. Cool for 5 minutes before serving.

Chicken Saltimbocca Sandwiches

Servings: 3
Cooking Time: 11 Minutes

Ingredients:
- 3 5- to 6-ounce boneless skinless chicken breasts
- 6 Thin prosciutto slices
- 6 Provolone cheese slices
- 3 Long soft rolls, such as hero, hoagie, or Italian sub rolls (gluten-free, if a concern), split open lengthwise
- 3 tablespoons Pesto, purchased or homemade (see the headnote)

Directions:
1. Preheat the air fryer to 400°F.
2. Wrap each chicken breast with 2 prosciutto slices, spiraling the prosciutto around the breast and overlapping the slices a bit to cover the breast. The prosciutto will stick to the chicken more readily than bacon does.
3. When the machine is at temperature, set the wrapped chicken breasts in the basket and air-fry undisturbed for 10 minutes, or until the prosciutto is frizzled and the chicken is cooked through.
4. Overlap 2 cheese slices on each breast. Air-fry undisturbed for 1 minute, or until melted. Take the basket out of the machine.
5. Smear the insides of the rolls with the pesto, then use kitchen tongs to put a wrapped and cheesy chicken breast in each roll.

White Bean Veggie Burgers

Servings: 3
Cooking Time: 13 Minutes

Ingredients:
- 1⅓ cups Drained and rinsed canned white beans
- 3 tablespoons Rolled oats (not quick-cooking or steel-cut; gluten-free, if a concern)
- 3 tablespoons Chopped walnuts
- 2 teaspoons Olive oil
- 2 teaspoons Lemon juice
- 1½ teaspoons Dijon mustard (gluten-free, if a concern)
- ¾ teaspoon Dried sage leaves
- ¼ teaspoon Table salt
- Olive oil spray
- 3 Whole-wheat buns or gluten-free whole-grain buns (if a concern), split open

Directions:
1. Preheat the air fryer to 400°F.
2. Place the beans, oats, walnuts, oil, lemon juice, mustard, sage, and salt in a food processor. Cover and process to make a coarse paste that will hold its shape, about like wet sugar-cookie dough, stopping the machine to scrape down the inside of the canister at least once.
3. Scrape down and remove the blade. With clean and wet hands, form the bean paste into two 4-inch patties for the small batch, three 4-inch patties for the medium, or four 4-inch patties for the large batch. Generously coat the patties on both sides with olive oil spray.
4. Set them in the basket with some space between them and air-fry undisturbed for 12 minutes, or until lightly brown and crisp at the edges. The tops of the burgers will feel firm to the touch.
5. Use a nonstick-safe spatula, and perhaps a flatware fork for balance, to transfer the burgers to a cutting board. Set the buns cut side down in the basket in one layer (working in batches as necessary) and air-fry undisturbed for 1 minute, to toast a bit and warm up. Serve the burgers warm in the buns.

Chicken Apple Brie Melt

Servings: 3
Cooking Time: 13 Minutes

Ingredients:
- 3 5- to 6-ounce boneless skinless chicken breasts
- Vegetable oil spray
- 1½ teaspoons Dried herbes de Provence
- 3 ounces Brie, rind removed, thinly sliced
- 6 Thin cored apple slices
- 3 French rolls (gluten-free, if a concern)
- 2 tablespoons Dijon mustard (gluten-free, if a concern)

Directions:
1. Preheat the air fryer to 375°F.
2. Lightly coat all sides of the chicken breasts with vegetable oil spray. Sprinkle the breasts evenly with the herbes de Provence.
3. When the machine is at temperature, set the breasts in the basket and air-fry undisturbed for 10 minutes.
4. Top the chicken breasts with the apple slices, then the cheese. Air-fry undisturbed for 2 minutes, or until the cheese is melty and bubbling.
5. Use a nonstick-safe spatula and kitchen tongs, for balance, to transfer the breasts to a cutting board. Set the rolls in the basket and air-fry for 1 minute to warm through. (Putting them in the machine without splitting them keeps the insides very soft while the outside gets a little crunchy.)
6. Transfer the rolls to the cutting board. Split them open lengthwise, then spread 1 teaspoon mustard on each cut side. Set a prepared chicken breast on the bottom of a roll and close with its top, repeating as necessary to make additional sandwiches. Serve warm.

Chicken Spiedies

Servings: 3
Cooking Time: 12 Minutes

Ingredients:
- 1¼ pounds Boneless skinless chicken thighs, trimmed of any fat blobs and cut into 2-inch pieces
- 3 tablespoons Red wine vinegar
- 2 tablespoons Olive oil
- 2 tablespoons Minced fresh mint leaves
- 2 tablespoons Minced fresh parsley leaves
- 2 teaspoons Minced fresh dill fronds
- ¾ teaspoon Fennel seeds
- ¾ teaspoon Table salt
- Up to a ¼ teaspoon Red pepper flakes
- 3 Long soft rolls, such as hero, hoagie, or Italian sub rolls (gluten-free, if a concern), split open lengthwise
- 4½ tablespoons Regular or low-fat mayonnaise (not fat-free; gluten-free, if a concern)
- 1½ tablespoons Distilled white vinegar
- 1½ teaspoons Ground black pepper

Directions:
1. Mix the chicken, vinegar, oil, mint, parsley, dill, fennel seeds, salt, and red pepper flakes in a zip-closed plastic bag. Seal, gently massage the marinade ingredients into the meat, and refrigerate for at least 2 hours or up to 6 hours. (Longer than that and the meat can turn rubbery.)
2. Set the plastic bag out on the counter (to make the contents a little less frigid). Preheat the air fryer to 400°F.
3. When the machine is at temperature, use kitchen tongs to set the chicken thighs in the basket (discard any remaining marinade) and air-fry undisturbed for 6 minutes. Turn the thighs over and continue air-frying undisturbed for 6 minutes more, until well browned, cooked through, and even a little crunchy.
4. Dump the contents of the basket onto a wire rack and cool for 2 or 3 minutes. Divide the chicken evenly between the rolls. Whisk the mayonnaise, vinegar, and black pepper in a small bowl until smooth. Drizzle this sauce over the chicken pieces in the rolls.

Perfect Burgers

Servings: 3
Cooking Time: 13 Minutes

Ingredients:
- 1 pound 2 ounces 90% lean ground beef
- 1½ tablespoons Worcestershire sauce (gluten-free, if a concern)
- ½ teaspoon Ground black pepper
- 3 Hamburger buns (gluten-free if a concern), split open

Directions:
1. Preheat the air fryer to 375°F .
2. Gently mix the ground beef, Worcestershire sauce, and pepper in a bowl until well combined but preserving as much of the meat's fibers as possible. Divide this mixture into two 5-inch patties for the small batch, three 5-inch patties for the medium, or four 5-inch patties for the large. Make a thumbprint indentation in the center of each patty, about halfway through the meat.
3. Set the patties in the basket in one layer with some space between them. Air-fry undisturbed for 10 minutes, or until an instant-read meat thermometer inserted into the center of a burger registers 160°F (a medium-well burger). You may need to add 2 minutes cooking time if the air fryer is at 360°F.
4. Use a nonstick-safe spatula, and perhaps a flatware fork for balance, to transfer the burgers to a cutting board. Set the buns cut side down in the basket in one layer (working in batches as necessary) and air-fry undisturbed for 1 minute, to toast a bit and warm up. Serve the burgers in the warm buns.

Sausage And Pepper Heros

Servings: 3
Cooking Time: 11 Minutes

Ingredients:
- 3 links (about 9 ounces total) Sweet Italian sausages (gluten-free, if a concern)
- 1½ Medium red or green bell pepper(s), stemmed, cored, and cut into ½-inch-wide strips
- 1 medium Yellow or white onion(s), peeled, halved, and sliced into thin half-moons
- 3 Long soft rolls, such as hero, hoagie, or Italian sub rolls (gluten-free, if a concern), split open lengthwise
- For garnishing Balsamic vinegar
- For garnishing Fresh basil leaves

Directions:
1. Preheat the air fryer to 400°F.
2. When the machine is at temperature, set the sausage links in the basket in one layer and air-fry undisturbed for 5 minutes.
3. Add the pepper strips and onions. Continue air-frying, tossing and rearranging everything about once every minute, for 5 minutes, or until the sausages are browned and an instant-read meat thermometer inserted into one of the links registers 160°F.
4. Use a nonstick-safe spatula and kitchen tongs to transfer the sausages and vegetables to a cutting board. Set the rolls cut side down in the basket in one layer (working in batches as necessary) and air-fry undisturbed for 1 minute, to toast the rolls a bit and warm them up. Set 1 sausage with some pepper strips and onions in each warm roll, sprinkle balsamic vinegar over the sandwich fillings, and garnish with basil leaves.

Eggplant Parmesan Subs

Servings: 2
Cooking Time: 13 Minutes

Ingredients:
- 4 Peeled eggplant slices (about ½ inch thick and 3 inches in diameter)
- Olive oil spray
- 2 tablespoons plus 2 teaspoons Jarred pizza sauce, any variety except creamy
- ¼ cup (about ⅔ ounce) Finely grated Parmesan cheese
- 2 Small, long soft rolls, such as hero, hoagie, or Italian sub rolls (gluten-free, if a concern), split open lengthwise

Directions:
1. Preheat the air fryer to 350°F .
2. When the machine is at temperature, coat both sides of the eggplant slices with olive oil spray. Set them in the basket in one layer and air-fry undisturbed for 10 minutes, until lightly browned and softened.
3. Increase the machine's temperature to 375°F (or 370°F, if that's the closest setting—unless the machine is already at 360°F, in which case leave it alone). Top each eggplant slice with 2 teaspoons pizza sauce, then 1 tablespoon cheese. Air-fry undisturbed for 2 minutes, or until the cheese has melted.
4. Use a nonstick-safe spatula, and perhaps a flatware fork for balance, to transfer the eggplant slices cheese side up to a cutting board. Set the roll(s) cut side down in the basket in one layer (working in batches as necessary) and air-fry undisturbed for 1 minute, to toast the rolls a bit and warm them up. Set 2 eggplant slices in each warm roll.

Dijon Thyme Burgers

Servings: 3
Cooking Time: 18 Minutes

Ingredients:
- 1 pound lean ground beef
- ⅓ cup panko breadcrumbs
- ¼ cup finely chopped onion
- 3 tablespoons Dijon mustard
- 1 tablespoon chopped fresh thyme
- 4 teaspoons Worcestershire sauce
- 1 teaspoon salt
- freshly ground black pepper
- Topping (optional):
- 2 tablespoons Dijon mustard
- 1 tablespoon dark brown sugar
- 1 teaspoon Worcestershire sauce
- 4 ounces sliced Swiss cheese, optional

Directions:
1. Combine all the burger ingredients together in a large bowl and mix well. Divide the meat into 4 equal portions and then form the burgers, being careful not to over-handle the meat. One good way to do this is to throw the meat back and forth from one hand to another, packing the meat each time you catch it. Flatten the balls into patties, making an indentation in the center of each patty with your thumb (this will help it stay flat as it cooks) and flattening the sides of the burgers so that they will fit nicely into the air fryer basket.
2. Preheat the air fryer to 370°F.
3. If you don't have room for all four burgers, air-fry two or three burgers at a time for 8 minutes. Flip the burgers over and air-fry for another 6 minutes.
4. While the burgers are cooking combine the Dijon mustard, dark brown sugar, and Worcestershire sauce in a small bowl and mix well. This optional topping to the burgers really adds a boost of flavor at the end. Spread the Dijon topping evenly on each burger. If you cooked the burgers in batches, return the first batch to the cooker at this time – it's ok to place the fourth burger on top of the others in the center of the basket. Air-fry the burgers for another 3 minutes.
5. Finally, if desired, top each burger with a slice of Swiss cheese. Lower the air fryer tem-

perature to 330°F and air-fry for another minute to melt the cheese. Serve the burgers on toasted brioche buns, dressed the way you like them.

Reuben Sandwiches

Servings: 2
Cooking Time: 11 Minutes

Ingredients:

- ½ pound Sliced deli corned beef
- 4 teaspoons Regular or low-fat mayonnaise (not fat-free)
- 4 Rye bread slices
- 2 tablespoons plus 2 teaspoons Russian dressing
- ½ cup Purchased sauerkraut, squeezed by the handful over the sink to get rid of excess moisture
- 2 ounces (2 to 4 slices) Swiss cheese slices (optional)

Directions:

1. Set the corned beef in the basket, slip the basket into the machine, and heat the air fryer to 400°F. Air-fry undisturbed for 3 minutes from the time the basket is put in the machine, just to warm up the meat.
2. Use kitchen tongs to transfer the corned beef to a cutting board. Spread 1 teaspoon mayonnaise on one side of each slice of rye bread, rubbing the mayonnaise into the bread with a small flatware knife.
3. Place the bread slices mayonnaise side down on a cutting board. Spread the Russian dressing over the "dry" side of each slice. For one sandwich, top one slice of bread with the corned beef, sauerkraut, and cheese (if using). For two sandwiches, top two slices of bread each with half of the corned beef, sauerkraut, and cheese (if using). Close the sandwiches with the remaining bread, setting it mayonnaise side up on top.
4. Set the sandwich(es) in the basket and air-fry undisturbed for 8 minutes, or until browned and crunchy.
5. Use a nonstick-safe spatula, and perhaps a flatware fork for balance, to transfer the sandwich(es) to a cutting board. Cool for 2 or 3 minutes before slicing in half and serving.

Chili Cheese Dogs

Servings: 3
Cooking Time: 12 Minutes

Ingredients:

- ¾ pound Lean ground beef
- 1½ tablespoons Chile powder
- 1 cup plus 2 tablespoons Jarred sofrito
- 3 Hot dogs (gluten-free, if a concern)
- 3 Hot dog buns (gluten-free, if a concern), split open lengthwise
- 3 tablespoons Finely chopped scallion
- 9 tablespoons (a little more than 2 ounces) Shredded Cheddar cheese

Directions:

1. Crumble the ground beef into a medium or large saucepan set over medium heat. Brown well, stirring often to break up the clumps. Add the chile powder and cook for 30 seconds, stirring the whole time. Stir in the sofrito and bring to a simmer. Reduce the heat to low and simmer, stirring occasionally, for 5 minutes. Keep warm.
2. Preheat the air fryer to 400°F.
3. When the machine is at temperature, put the hot dogs in the basket and air-fry undisturbed for 10 minutes, or until the hot dogs are bubbling and blistered, even a little crisp.
4. Use kitchen tongs to put the hot dogs in the buns. Top each with a ½ cup of the ground beef mixture, 1 tablespoon of the minced scallion, and 3 tablespoons of the cheese. (The scallion should go under the cheese so it superheats and wilts a bit.) Set the filled hot dog buns in the basket and air-fry undisturbed for 2 minutes, or until the cheese has melted.
5. Remove the basket from the machine. Cool the chili cheese dogs in the basket for 5 minutes before serving.

Fish And Seafood Recipes

Cajun Flounder Fillets 85
Crabmeat-stuffed Flounder 85
Tuna Patties With Dill Sauce 85
Basil Crab Cakes With Fresh Salad...................................86
Sweet & Spicy Swordfish Kebabs.....................................86
Catfish Nuggets 87
Tex-mex Fish Tacos 87
Cheese & Crab Stuffed Mushrooms 87
Mediterranean Salmon Burgers 88
Salmon Puttanesca En Papillotte With Zucchini 88
Peppery Tilapia Roulade..88
Holliday Lobster Salad 89
Rich Salmon Burgers With Broccoli Slaw 89
Tuscan Salmon 89
Sesame-crusted Tuna Steaks...90
Home-style Fish Sticks 90
Citrus Baked Scallops..90
Shrimp Patties...90
Coconut-shrimp Po' Boys 91
Lemony Tuna Steaks 91
Easy-peasy Shrimp...91
Nutty Shrimp With Amaretto Glaze 92
Fish Sticks For Kids 92
Stuffed Shrimp Wrapped In Bacon 92
Collard Green & Cod Packets..93
Feta & Shrimp Pita...93
Crunchy Clam Strips...93

Cajun Flounder Fillets

Servings: 2
Cooking Time: 5 Minutes

Ingredients:
- 2 4-ounce skinless flounder fillet(s)
- 2 teaspoons Peanut oil
- 1 teaspoon Purchased or homemade Cajun dried seasoning blend (see the headnote)

Directions:
1. Preheat the air fryer to 400°F.
2. Oil the fillet(s) by drizzling on the peanut oil, then gently rubbing in the oil with your clean, dry fingers. Sprinkle the seasoning blend evenly over both sides of the fillet(s).
3. When the machine is at temperature, set the fillet(s) in the basket. If working with more than one fillet, they should not touch, although they may be quite close together, depending on the basket's size. Air-fry undisturbed for 5 minutes, or until lightly browned and cooked through.
4. Use a nonstick-safe spatula to transfer the fillets to a serving platter or plate(s). Serve at once.

Crabmeat-stuffed Flounder

Servings: 3
Cooking Time: 12 Minutes

Ingredients:
- 4½ ounces Purchased backfin or claw crabmeat, picked over for bits of shell and cartilage
- 6 Saltine crackers, crushed into fine crumbs
- 2 tablespoons plus 1 teaspoon Regular or low-fat mayonnaise (not fat-free)
- ¾ teaspoon Yellow prepared mustard
- 1½ teaspoons Worcestershire sauce
- ⅛ teaspoon Celery salt
- 3 5- to 6-ounce skinless flounder fillets
- Vegetable oil spray
- Mild paprika

Directions:
1. Preheat the air fryer to 400°F.
2. Gently mix the crabmeat, crushed saltines, mayonnaise, mustard, Worcestershire sauce, and celery salt in a bowl until well combined.
3. Generously coat the flat side of a fillet with vegetable oil spray. Set the fillet sprayed side down on your work surface. Cut the fillet in half widthwise, then cut one of the halves in half lengthwise. Set a scant ⅓ cup of the crabmeat mixture on top of the undivided half of the fish fillet, mounding the mixture to make an oval that somewhat fits the shape of the fillet with at least a ¼-inch border of fillet beyond the filling all around.
4. Take the two thin divided quarters (that is, the halves of the half) and lay them lengthwise over the filling, overlapping at each end and leaving a little space in the middle where the filling peeks through. Coat the top of the stuffed flounder piece with vegetable oil spray, then sprinkle paprika over the stuffed flounder fillet. Set aside and use the remaining fillet(s) to make more stuffed flounder "packets," repeating steps 3 and
5. Use a nonstick-safe spatula to transfer the stuffed flounder fillets to the basket. Leave as much space between them as possible. Air-fry undisturbed for 12 minutes, or until lightly brown and firm (but not hard).
6. Use that same spatula, plus perhaps another one, to transfer the fillets to a serving platter or plates. Cool for a minute or two, then serve hot.

Tuna Patties With Dill Sauce

Servings: 6
Cooking Time: 10 Minutes

Ingredients:
- Two 5-ounce cans albacore tuna, drained
- ½ teaspoon garlic powder
- 2 teaspoons dried dill, divided
- ½ teaspoon black pepper
- ½ teaspoon salt, divided
- ¼ cup minced onion
- 1 large egg

- 7 tablespoons mayonnaise, divided
- ¼ cup panko breadcrumbs
- 1 teaspoon fresh lemon juice
- ¼ teaspoon fresh lemon zest
- 6 pieces butterleaf lettuce
- 1 cup diced tomatoes

Directions:

1. In a large bowl, mix the tuna with the garlic powder, 1 teaspoon of the dried dill, the black pepper, ¼ teaspoon of the salt, and the onion. Make sure to use the back of a fork to really break up the tuna so there are no large chunks.

2. Mix in the egg and 1 tablespoon of the mayonnaise; then fold in the breadcrumbs so the tuna begins to form a thick batter that holds together.

3. Portion the tuna mixture into 6 equal patties and place on a plate lined with parchment paper in the refrigerator for at least 30 minutes. This will help the patties hold together in the air fryer.

4. When ready to cook, preheat the air fryer to 350°F.

5. Liberally spray the metal trivet that sits inside the air fryer basket with olive oil mist and place the patties onto the trivet.

6. Cook for 5 minutes, flip, and cook another 5 minutes.

7. While the patties are cooking, make the dill sauce by combining the remaining 6 tablespoons of mayonnaise with the remaining 1 teaspoon of dill, the lemon juice, the lemon zest, and the remaining ¼ teaspoon of salt. Set aside.

8. Remove the patties from the air fryer.

9. Place 1 slice of lettuce on a plate and top with the tuna patty and a tomato slice. Repeat to form the remaining servings. Drizzle the dill dressing over the top. Serve immediately.

Basil Crab Cakes With Fresh Salad

Servings: 2
Cooking Time: 25 Minutes

Ingredients:
- 8 oz lump crabmeat
- 2 tbsp mayonnaise
- ½ tsp Dijon mustard
- ½ tsp lemon juice
- ½ tsp lemon zest
- 2 tsp minced yellow onion
- ¼ tsp prepared horseradish
- ¼ cup flour
- 1 egg white, beaten
- 1 tbsp basil, minced
- 1 tbsp olive oil
- 2 tsp white wine vinegar
- Salt and pepper to taste
- 4 oz arugula
- ½ cup blackberries
- ¼ cup pine nuts
- 2 lemon wedges

Directions:

1. Preheat air fryer to 400°F. Combine the crabmeat, mayonnaise, mustard, lemon juice and zest, onion, horseradish, flour, egg white, and basil in a bowl. Form mixture into 4 patties. Place the patties in the lightly greased frying basket and Air Fry for 10 minutes, flipping once. Combine olive oil, vinegar, salt, and pepper in a bowl. Toss in the arugula and share into 2 medium bowls. Add 2 crab cakes to each bowl and scatter with blackberries, pine nuts, and lemon wedges. Serve warm.

Sweet & Spicy Swordfish Kebabs

Servings: 4
Cooking Time: 30 Minutes

Ingredients:
- ½ cup canned pineapple chunks, drained, juice reserved
- 1 lb swordfish steaks, cubed
- ½ cup large red grapes
- 1 tbsp honey
- 2 tsp grated fresh ginger
- 1 tsp olive oil
- Pinch cayenne pepper

Directions:

1. Preheat air fryer to 370°F. Poke 8 bamboo skewers through the swordfish, pineapple, and grapes. Mix the honey, 1 tbsp of pineapple juice, ginger, olive oil, and cayenne in a bowl, then use a brush to rub the mix on the kebabs. Allow the marinate to sit on the kebab for 10 minutes. Grill the kebabs for 8-12 minutes until the fish is cooked through and the fruit is soft and glazed. Brush the kebabs again with the mix, then toss the rest of the marinade. Serve warm and enjoy!

Catfish Nuggets

Servings: 4
Cooking Time: 7 Minutes Per Batch

Ingredients:
- 2 medium catfish fillets, cut in chunks (approximately 1 x 2 inch)
- salt and pepper
- 2 eggs
- 2 tablespoons skim milk
- ½ cup cornstarch
- 1 cup panko breadcrumbs, crushed
- oil for misting or cooking spray

Directions:
1. Season catfish chunks with salt and pepper to your liking.
2. Beat together eggs and milk in a small bowl.
3. Place cornstarch in a second small bowl.
4. Place breadcrumbs in a third small bowl.
5. Dip catfish chunks in cornstarch, dip in egg wash, shake off excess, then roll in breadcrumbs.
6. Spray all sides of catfish chunks with oil or cooking spray.
7. Place chunks in air fryer basket in a single layer, leaving space between for air circulation.
8. Cook at 390°F for 4minutes, turn, and cook an additional 3 minutes, until fish flakes easily and outside is crispy brown.
9. Repeat steps 7 and 8 to cook remaining catfish nuggets.

Tex-mex Fish Tacos

Servings:3
Cooking Time: 7 Minutes

Ingredients:
- ¾ teaspoon Chile powder
- ¼ teaspoon Ground cumin
- ¼ teaspoon Dried oregano
- 3 5-ounce skinless mahi-mahi fillets
- Vegetable oil spray
- 3 Corn or flour tortillas
- 6 tablespoons Diced tomatoes
- 3 tablespoons Regular, low-fat, or fat-free sour cream

Directions:
1. Preheat the air fryer to 400°F.
2. Stir the chile powder, cumin, and oregano in a small bowl until well combined.
3. Coat each piece of fish all over (even the sides and ends) with vegetable oil spray. Sprinkle the spice mixture evenly over all sides of the fillets. Lightly spray them again.
4. When the machine is at temperature, set the fillets in the basket with as much air space between them as possible. Air-fry undisturbed for 7 minutes, until lightly browned and firm but not hard.
5. Use a nonstick-safe spatula to transfer the fillets to a wire rack. Microwave the tortillas on high for a few seconds, until supple. Put a fillet in each tortilla and top each with 2 tablespoons diced tomatoes and 1 tablespoon sour cream.

Cheese & Crab Stuffed Mushrooms

Servings: 2
Cooking Time: 30 Minutes

Ingredients:
- 6 oz lump crabmeat, shells discarded
- 6 oz mascarpone cheese, softened
- 2 jalapeño peppers, minced
- ¼ cup diced red onions
- 2 tsp grated Parmesan cheese
- 2 portobello mushroom caps
- 2 tbsp butter, divided
- ½ tsp prepared horseradish
- ¼ tsp Worcestershire sauce
- ¼ tsp smoked paprika
- Salt and pepper to taste
- ¼ cup bread crumbs

Directions:
1. Melt 1 tbsp of butter in a skillet over heat for 30 seconds. Add in onion and cook for 3 minutes until tender. Stir in mascarpone cheese, Parmesan cheese, horseradish, jalapeño peppers, Worcestershire sauce, paprika, salt and pepper and cook for 2 minutes until smooth. Fold in crabmeat. Spoon mixture into mushroom caps. Set aside.
2. Preheat air fryer at 350°F. Microwave the remaining butter until melted. Stir in breadcrumbs. Scatter over stuffed mushrooms. Place mushrooms in the greased frying basket and Bake for 8 minutes. Serve immediately.

Mediterranean Salmon Burgers

Servings: 4
Cooking Time: 30 Minutes

Ingredients:
- 1 lb salmon fillets
- 1 scallion, diced
- 4 tbsp mayonnaise
- 1 egg
- 1 tsp capers, drained
- Salt and pepper to taste
- ¼ tsp paprika
- 1 lemon, zested
- 1 lemon, sliced
- 1 tbsp chopped dill
- ¼ cup bread crumbs
- 4 buns, toasted
- 4 tsp whole-grain mustard
- 4 lettuce leaves
- 1 small tomato, sliced

Directions:
1. Preheat air fryer to 400°F. Divide salmon in half. Cut one of the halves into chunks and transfer the chunks to the food processor. Also, add scallion, 2 tablespoons mayonnaise, egg, capers, dill, salt, pepper, paprika, and lemon zest. Pulse to puree. Dice the rest of the salmon into ¼-inch chunks. Combine chunks and puree along with bread crumbs in a large bowl. Shape the fish into 4 patties and transfer to the frying basket. Air Fry for 5 minutes, then flip the patties. Air Fry for another 5 to 7 minutes. Place the patties each on a bun along with 1 teaspoon mustard, mayonnaise, lettuce, lemon slices, and a slice of tomato. Serve and enjoy.

Salmon Puttanesca En Papillotte With Zucchini

Servings: 2
Cooking Time: 17 Minutes

Ingredients:
- 1 small zucchini, sliced into ¼-inch thick half moons
- 1 teaspoon olive oil
- salt and freshly ground black pepper
- 2 (5-ounce) salmon fillets
- 1 beefsteak tomato, chopped (about 1 cup)
- 1 tablespoon capers, rinsed
- 10 black olives, pitted and sliced
- 2 tablespoons dry vermouth or white wine 2 tablespoons butter
- ¼ cup chopped fresh basil, chopped

Directions:
1. Preheat the air fryer to 400°F.
2. Toss the zucchini with the olive oil, salt and freshly ground black pepper. Transfer the zucchini into the air fryer basket and air-fry for 5 minutes, shaking the basket once or twice during the cooking process.
3. Cut out 2 large rectangles of parchment paper – about 13-inches by 15-inches each. Divide the air-fried zucchini between the two pieces of parchment paper, placing the vegetables in the center of each rectangle.
4. Place a fillet of salmon on each pile of zucchini. Season the fish very well with salt and pepper. Toss the tomato, capers, olives and vermouth (or white wine) together in a bowl. Divide the tomato mixture between the two fish packages, placing it on top of the fish fillets and pouring any juice out of the bowl onto the fish. Top each fillet with a tablespoon of butter.
5. Fold up each parchment square. Bring two edges together and fold them over a few times, leaving some space above the fish. Twist the open sides together and upwards so they can serve as handles for the packet, but don't let them extend beyond the top of the air fryer basket.
6. Place the two packages into the air fryer and air-fry at 400°F for 12 minutes. The packages should be puffed up and slightly browned when fully cooked. Once cooked, let the fish sit in the parchment for 2 minutes.
7. Serve the fish in the parchment paper, or if desired, remove the parchment paper before serving. Garnish with a little fresh basil.

Peppery Tilapia Roulade

Servings: 4
Cooking Time: 25 Minutes

Ingredients:
- 4 jarred roasted red pepper slices
- 1 egg
- ½ cup breadcrumbs
- Salt and pepper to taste

- 4 tilapia fillets
- 2 tbsp butter, melted
- 4 lime wedges
- 1 tsp dill

Directions:

1. Preheat air fryer at 350°F. Beat the egg and 2 tbsp of water in a bowl. In another bowl, mix the breadcrumbs, salt, and pepper. Place a red pepper slice and sprinkle with dill on each fish fillet. Tightly roll tilapia fillets from one short end to the other. Secure with toothpicks. Roll each fillet in the egg mixture, then dredge them in the breadcrumbs. Place fish rolls in the greased frying basket and drizzle the tops with melted butter. Roast for 6 minutes. Let rest in a serving dish for 5 minutes before removing the toothpicks. Serve with lime wedges. Enjoy!

Holliday Lobster Salad

Servings: 2
Cooking Time: 20 Minutes

Ingredients:

- 2 lobster tails
- ¼ cup mayonnaise
- 2 tsp lemon juice
- 1 stalk celery, sliced
- 2 tsp chopped chives
- 2 tsp chopped tarragon
- Salt and pepper to taste
- 2 tomato slices
- 4 cucumber slices
- 1 avocado, diced

Directions:

1. Preheat air fryer to 400°F. Using kitchen shears, cut down the middle of each lobster tail on the softer side. Carefully run your finger between the lobster meat and the shell to loosen meat. Place lobster tails, cut sides up, in the frying basket, and Air Fry for 8 minutes. Transfer to a large plate and let cool for 3 minutes until easy to handle, then pull lobster meat from the shell and roughly chop it. Combine chopped lobster, mayonnaise, lemon juice, celery, chives, tarragon, salt, and pepper in a bowl. Divide between 2 medium plates and top with tomato slices, cucumber and avocado cubes. Serve immediately.

Rich Salmon Burgers With Broccoli Slaw

Servings: 4
Cooking Time: 25 Minutes

Ingredients:

- 1 lb salmon fillets
- 1 egg
- ¼ cup dill, chopped
- 1 cup bread crumbs
- Salt to taste
- ½ tsp cayenne pepper
- 1 lime, zested
- 1 tsp fish sauce
- 4 buns
- 3 cups chopped broccoli
- ½ cup shredded carrots
- ¼ cup sunflower seeds
- 2 garlic cloves, minced
- 1 cup Greek yogurt

Directions:

1. Preheat air fryer to 360°F. Blitz the salmon fillets in your food processor until they are finely chopped. Remove to a large bowl and add egg, dill, bread crumbs, salt, and cayenne. Stir to combine. Form the mixture into 4 patties. Put them into the frying basket and Bake for 10 minutes, flipping once. Combine broccoli, carrots, sunflower seeds, garlic, salt, lime, fish sauce, and Greek yogurt in a bowl. Serve the salmon burgers onto buns with broccoli slaw. Enjoy!

Tuscan Salmon

Servings: 4
Cooking Time: 15 Minutes

Ingredients:

- 2 tbsp olive oil
- 4 salmon fillets
- ½ tsp salt
- ¼ tsp red pepper flakes
- 1 tsp chopped dill
- 2 tomatoes, diced
- ¼ cup sliced black olives
- 4 lemon slices

Directions:

1. Preheat air fryer to 380°F. Lightly brush the olive oil on both sides of the salmon fillets and

season them with salt, red flakes, and dill. Put the fillets in a single layer in the frying basket, then layer the tomatoes and black olives over the top. Top each fillet with a lemon slice. Bake for 8 minutes. Serve and enjoy!

Sesame-crusted Tuna Steaks

Servings: 3
Cooking Time: 10-13 Minutes

Ingredients:
- ½ cup Sesame seeds, preferably a blend of white and black
- 1½ tablespoons Toasted sesame oil
- 3 6-ounce skinless tuna steaks

Directions:
1. Preheat the air fryer to 400°F.
2. Pour the sesame seeds on a dinner plate. Use ½ tablespoon of the sesame oil as a rub on both sides and the edges of a tuna steak. Set it in the sesame seeds, then turn it several times, pressing gently, to create an even coating of the seeds, including around the steak's edge. Set aside and continue coating the remaining steak(s).
3. When the machine is at temperature, set the steaks in the basket with as much air space between them as possible. Air-fry undisturbed for 10 minutes for medium-rare (not USDA-approved), or 12 to 13 minutes for cooked through (USDA-approved).
4. Use a nonstick-safe spatula to transfer the steaks to serving plates. Serve hot.

Home-style Fish Sticks

Servings: 4
Cooking Time: 30 Minutes

Ingredients:
- 1 lb cod fillets, cut into sticks
- 1 cup flour
- 1 egg
- ¼ cup cornmeal
- Salt and pepper to taste
- ¼ tsp smoked paprika
- 1 lemon

Directions:
1. Preheat air fryer at 350°F. In a bowl, add ½ cup of flour. In another bowl, beat the egg and

in a third bowl, combine the remaining flour, cornmeal, salt, black pepper and paprika. Roll the sticks in the flour, shake off excess flour. Then, dip them in the egg, shake off excess egg. Finally, dredge them in the cornmeal mixture. Place fish fingers in the greased frying basket and Air Fry for 10 minutes, flipping once. Serve with squeezed lemon.

Citrus Baked Scallops

Servings: 4
Cooking Time: 15 Minutes

Ingredients:
- 1 tsp lemon juice
- 1 tsp lime juice
- 2 tsp olive oil
- Salt and pepper to taste
- 1 lb sea scallops
- 2 tbsp chives, chopped

Directions:
1. Preheat air fryer to 390°F. Combine lemon and lime juice, olive oil, salt, and pepper in a bowl. Toss in scallops to coat. Place the scallops in the greased frying basket and Bake for 5 -8 minutes, tossing once halfway through, until the scallops are just firm to the touch. Serve topped with chives and enjoy!

Shrimp Patties

Servings: 4
Cooking Time: 10 Minutes

Ingredients:
- ½ pound shelled and deveined raw shrimp
- ¼ cup chopped red bell pepper
- ¼ cup chopped green onion
- ¼ cup chopped celery
- 2 cups cooked sushi rice
- ½ teaspoon garlic powder
- ½ teaspoon Old Bay Seasoning
- ½ teaspoon salt
- 2 teaspoons Worcestershire sauce
- ½ cup plain breadcrumbs
- oil for misting or cooking spray

Directions:
1. Finely chop the shrimp. You can do this in a food processor, but it takes only a few pulses. Be careful not to overprocess into mush.

2. Place shrimp in a large bowl and add all other ingredients except the breadcrumbs and oil. Stir until well combined.

3. Preheat air fryer to 390°F.

4. Shape shrimp mixture into 8 patties, no more than ½-inch thick. Roll patties in breadcrumbs and mist with oil or cooking spray.

5. Place 4 shrimp patties in air fryer basket and cook at 390°F for 10 minutes, until shrimp cooks through and outside is crispy.

6. Repeat step 5 to cook remaining shrimp patties.

Coconut-shrimp Po' Boys

Servings: 4
Cooking Time: 5 Minutes

Ingredients:
- ½ cup cornstarch
- 2 eggs
- 2 tablespoons milk
- ¾ cup shredded coconut
- ½ cup panko breadcrumbs
- 1 pound (31-35 count) shrimp, peeled and deveined
- Old Bay Seasoning
- oil for misting or cooking spray
- 2 large hoagie rolls
- honey mustard or light mayonnaise
- 1½ cups shredded lettuce
- 1 large tomato, thinly sliced

Directions:
1. Place cornstarch in a shallow dish or plate.

2. In another shallow dish, beat together eggs and milk.

3. In a third dish mix the coconut and panko crumbs.

4. Sprinkle shrimp with Old Bay Seasoning to taste.

5. Dip shrimp in cornstarch to coat lightly, dip in egg mixture, shake off excess, and roll in coconut mixture to coat well.

6. Spray both sides of coated shrimp with oil or cooking spray.

7. Cook half the shrimp in a single layer at 390°F for 5minutes.

8. Repeat to cook remaining shrimp.

9. To Assemble

10. Split each hoagie lengthwise, leaving one long edge intact.

11. Place in air fryer basket and cook at 390°F for 1 to 2minutes or until heated through.

12. Remove buns, break apart, and place on 4 plates, cut side up.

13. Spread with honey mustard and/or mayonnaise.

14. Top with shredded lettuce, tomato slices, and coconut shrimp.

Lemony Tuna Steaks

Servings: 4
Cooking Time: 20 Minutes

Ingredients:
- ½ tbsp olive oil
- 1 garlic clove, minced
- Salt to taste
- ¼ tsp jalapeno powder
- 1 tbsp lemon juice
- 1 tbsp chopped cilantro
- ½ tbsp chopped dill
- 4 tuna steaks
- 1 lemon, thinly sliced

Directions:
1. Stir olive oil, garlic, salt, jalapeno powder, lemon juice, and cilantro in a wide bowl. Coat the tuna on all sides in the mixture. Cover and marinate for at least 20 minutes

2. Preheat air fryer to 380°F. Arrange the tuna on a single layer in the greased frying basket and throw out the excess marinade. Bake for 6-8 minutes. Remove the basket and let the tuna rest in it for 5 minutes. Transfer to plates and garnish with lemon slices. Serve sprinkled with dill.

Easy-peasy Shrimp

Servings:2
Cooking Time: 15 Minutes

Ingredients:
- 1 lb tail-on shrimp, deveined
- 2 tbsp butter, melted
- 1 tbsp lemon juice
- 1 tbsp dill, chopped

Directions:
1. Preheat air fryer to 350ºF. Combine shrimp and butter in a bowl. Place shrimp in the

greased frying basket and Air Fry for 6 minutes, flipping once. Squeeze lemon juice over and top with dill. Serve hot.

Nutty Shrimp With Amaretto Glaze

Servings: 10
Cooking Time: 10 Minutes

Ingredients:
- 1 cup flour
- ½ teaspoon baking powder
- 1 teaspoon salt
- 2 eggs, beaten
- ½ cup milk
- 2 tablespoons olive or vegetable oil
- 2 cups sliced almonds
- 2 pounds large shrimp (about 32 to 40 shrimp), peeled and deveined, tails left on
- 2 cups amaretto liqueur

Directions:
1. Combine the flour, baking powder and salt in a large bowl. Add the eggs, milk and oil and stir until it forms a smooth batter. Coarsely crush the sliced almonds into a second shallow dish with your hands.
2. Dry the shrimp well with paper towels. Dip the shrimp into the batter and shake off any excess batter, leaving just enough to lightly coat the shrimp. Transfer the shrimp to the dish with the almonds and coat completely. Place the coated shrimp on a plate or baking sheet and when all the shrimp have been coated, freeze the shrimp for an 1 hour, or as long as a week before air-frying.
3. Preheat the air fryer to 400°F.
4. Transfer 8 frozen shrimp at a time to the air fryer basket. Air-fry for 6 minutes. Turn the shrimp over and air-fry for an additional 4 minutes. Repeat with the remaining shrimp.
5. While the shrimp are cooking, bring the Amaretto to a boil in a small saucepan on the stovetop. Lower the heat and simmer until it has reduced and thickened into a glaze – about 10 minutes.
6. Remove the shrimp from the air fryer and brush both sides with the warm amaretto glaze. Serve warm.

Fish Sticks For Kids

Servings: 8
Cooking Time: 6 Minutes

Ingredients:
- 8 ounces fish fillets (pollock or cod)
- salt (optional)
- ½ cup plain breadcrumbs
- oil for misting or cooking spray

Directions:
1. Cut fish fillets into "fingers" about ½ x 3 inches. Sprinkle with salt to taste, if desired.
2. Roll fish in breadcrumbs. Spray all sides with oil or cooking spray.
3. Place in air fryer basket in single layer and cook at 390°F for 6 minutes, until golden brown and crispy.

Stuffed Shrimp Wrapped In Bacon

Servings:4
Cooking Time: 30 Minutes

Ingredients:
- 1 lb shrimp, deveined and shelled
- 3 tbsp crumbled goat cheese
- 2 tbsp panko bread crumbs
- ¼ tsp soy sauce
- ½ tsp prepared horseradish
- ¼ tsp garlic powder
- ½ tsp chili powder
- 2 tsp mayonnaise
- Black pepper to taste
- 5 slices bacon, quartered
- ¼ cup chopped parsley

Directions:
1. Preheat air fryer to 400ºF. Butterfly shrimp by cutting down the spine of each shrimp without going all the way through. Combine the goat cheese, bread crumbs, soy sauce, horseradish, garlic powder, chili powder, mayonnaise, and black pepper in a bowl. Evenly press goat cheese mixture into shrimp. Wrap a piece of bacon around each piece of shrimp to hold in the cheese mixture. Place them in the frying basket and Air Fry for 8-10 minutes, flipping once. Top with parsley to serve.

Collard Green & Cod Packets

Servings: 4
Cooking Time: 20 Minutes

Ingredients:

- 2 cups collard greens, chopped
- 1 tsp salt
- ½ tsp dried rosemary
- ½ tsp dried thyme
- ½ tsp garlic powder
- 4 cod fillets
- 1 shallot, thinly sliced
- ¼ cup olive oil
- 1 lemon, juiced

Directions:

1. Preheat air fryer to 380°F. Mix together the salt, rosemary, thyme, and garlic powder in a small bowl. Rub the spice mixture onto the cod fillets. Divide the fish fillets among 4 sheets of foil. Top with shallot slices and collard greens. Drizzle with olive oil and lemon juice. Fold and seal the sides of the foil packets and then place them into the frying basket. Steam in the fryer for 11-13 minutes until the cod is cooked through. Serve and enjoy!

Feta & Shrimp Pita

Servings: 4
Cooking Time: 15 Minutes

Ingredients:

- 1 lb peeled shrimp, deveined
- 2 tbsp olive oil
- 1 tsp dried oregano
- ½ tsp dried thyme
- ½ tsp garlic powder
- ¼ tsp shallot powder
- ¼ tsp tarragon powder
- Salt and pepper to taste
- 4 whole-wheat pitas
- 4 oz feta cheese, crumbled
- 1 cup grated lettuce
- 1 tomato, diced
- ¼ cup black olives, sliced
- 1 lemon

Directions:

1. Preheat the oven to 380°F. Mix the shrimp with olive oil, oregano, thyme, garlic powder, shallot powder, tarragon powder salt, and pep-per in a bowl. Pour shrimp in a single layer in the frying basket and Bake for 6-8 minutes or until no longer pink and cooked through. Divide the shrimp into warmed pitas with feta, lettuce, tomato, olives, and a squeeze of lemon. Serve and enjoy!

Crunchy Clam Strips

Servings: 3
Cooking Time: 8 Minutes

Ingredients:

- ½ pound Clam strips, drained
- 1 Large egg, well beaten
- ½ cup All-purpose flour
- ½ cup Yellow cornmeal
- 1½ teaspoons Table salt
- 1½ teaspoons Ground black pepper
- Up to ¾ teaspoon Cayenne
- Vegetable oil spray

Directions:

1. Preheat the air fryer to 400°F.
2. Toss the clam strips and beaten egg in a bowl until the clams are well coated.
3. Mix the flour, cornmeal, salt, pepper, and cayenne in a large zip-closed plastic bag until well combined. Using a flatware fork or small kitchen tongs, lift the clam strips one by one out of the egg, letting any excess egg slip back into the rest. Put the strips in the bag with the flour mixture. Once all the strips are in the bag, seal it and shake gently until the strips are well coated.
4. Use kitchen tongs to pick out the clam strips and lay them on a cutting board (leaving any extra flour mixture in the bag to be discarded). Coat the strips on both sides with vegetable oil spray.
5. When the machine is at temperature, spread the clam strips in the basket in one layer. They may touch in places, but try to leave as much air space as possible around them. Air-fry undisturbed for 8 minutes, or until brown and crunchy.
6. Gently dump the contents of the basket onto a serving platter. Cool for just a minute or two before serving hot.

Desserts And Sweets Recipes

Apple Dumplings...95
Easy Bread Pudding 95
Homemade Chips Ahoy 95
Apple Crisp 96
Fried Cannoli Wontons 96
Fall Caramelized Apples 96
Peanut Butter S'mores..97
Coconut Crusted Bananas With Pineapple Sauce 97
Chocolate Rum Brownies 97
Bananas Foster Bread Pudding..98
White Chocolate Cranberry Blondies................................98
Choco-granola Bars With Cranberries..............................98
Cinnamon Tortilla Crisps 99
Coconut Cream Roll-ups...99
Fried Banana S'mores 99
Mixed Berry Pie..99
Nutty Cookies...100
Cherry Cheesecake Rolls 100
Cherry Hand Pies...100
Date Oat Cookies...101
Pear And Almond Biscotti Crumble 101
Mango Cobbler With Raspberries...................................101
Vegan Brownie Bites..102
Maple Cinnamon Cheesecake..102
Nutty Banana Bread...102
Vanilla Butter Cake 103
Baked Caramelized Peaches..103

Apple Dumplings

Servings: 4
Cooking Time: 25 Minutes

Ingredients:
- 1 Basic Pie Dough (see the following recipe)
- 4 medium Granny Smith or Pink Lady apples, peeled and cored
- 4 tablespoons sugar
- 4 teaspoons cinnamon
- ½ teaspoon ground nutmeg
- 4 tablespoons unsalted butter, melted
- 4 scoops ice cream, for serving

Directions:
1. Preheat the air fryer to 330°F.
2. Bring the pie crust recipe to room temperature.
3. Place the pie crust on a floured surface. Divide the dough into 4 equal pieces. Roll out each piece to ¼-inch-thick rounds. Place an apple onto each dough round. Sprinkle 1 tablespoon of sugar in the core part of each apple; sprinkle 1 teaspoon cinnamon and ⅛ teaspoon nutmeg over each. Place 1 tablespoon of butter into the center of each. Fold up the sides and fully cover the cored apples.
4. Place the dumplings into the air fryer basket and spray with cooking spray. Cook for 25 minutes. Check after 14 minutes cooking; if they're getting too brown, reduce the heat to 320°F and complete the cooking.
5. Serve hot apple dumplings with a scoop of ice cream.

Easy Bread Pudding

Servings: 4
Cooking Time: 25 Minutes

Ingredients:
- 2 cups sandwich bread cubes
- ½ cup pecan pieces
- ½ cup raisins
- 3 eggs
- ¼ cup half-and-half
- ¼ cup dark corn syrup
- 1 tsp vanilla extract
- 2 tbsp bourbon
- 2 tbsp dark brown sugar
- ¼ tsp ground cinnamon
- ½ tsp nutmeg
- ¼ tsp salt

Directions:
1. Preheat air fryer at 325°F. Spread the bread pieces in a cake pan and layer pecan pieces and raisins over the top. Whisk the eggs, half-and-half, corn syrup, bourbon, vanilla extract, sugar, cinnamon, nutmeg, and salt in a bowl. Pour egg mixture over pecan pieces. Let sit for 10 minutes. Place the cake pan in the frying basket and Bake for 15 minutes. Let cool onto a cooling rack for 10 minutes before slicing. Serve immediately.

Homemade Chips Ahoy

Servings: 4
Cooking Time: 20 Minutes

Ingredients:
- 1 tbsp coconut oil, melted
- 1 tbsp honey
- 1 tbsp milk
- ½ tsp vanilla extract
- ¼ cup oat flour
- 2 tbsp coconut sugar
- ¼ tsp salt
- ¼ tsp baking powder
- 2 tbsp chocolate chips

Directions:
1. Combine the coconut oil, honey, milk, and vanilla in a bowl. Add the oat flour, coconut sugar, salt, and baking powder. Stir until combined. Add the chocolate chips and stir. Preheat air fryer to 350°F. Pour the batter into a greased baking pan, leaving a little room in between. Bake for 7 minutes or until golden. Do not overcook. Move to a cooling rack and serve chilled.

Apple Crisp

Servings: 4
Cooking Time: 16 Minutes

Ingredients:
- Filling
- 3 Granny Smith apples, thinly sliced (about 4 cups)
- ¼ teaspoon ground cinnamon
- ⅛ teaspoon salt
- 1½ teaspoons lemon juice
- 2 tablespoons honey
- 1 tablespoon brown sugar
- cooking spray
- Crumb Topping
- 2 tablespoons oats
- 2 tablespoons oat bran
- 2 tablespoons cooked quinoa
- 2 tablespoons chopped walnuts
- 2 tablespoons brown sugar
- 2 teaspoons coconut oil

Directions:
1. Combine all filling ingredients and stir well so that apples are evenly coated.
2. Spray air fryer baking pan with nonstick cooking spray and spoon in the apple mixture.
3. Cook at 360°F for 5minutes. Stir well, scooping up from the bottom to mix apples and sauce.
4. At this point, the apples should be crisp-tender. Continue cooking in 3-minute intervals until apples are as soft as you like.
5. While apples are cooking, combine all topping ingredients in a small bowl. Stir until coconut oil mixes in well and distributes evenly. If your coconut oil is cold, it may be easier to mix in by hand.
6. When apples are cooked to your liking, sprinkle crumb mixture on top. Cook at 360°F for 8 minutes or until crumb topping is golden brown and crispy.

Fried Cannoli Wontons

Servings: 10
Cooking Time: 8 Minutes

Ingredients:
- 8 ounces Neufchâtel cream cheese
- ¼ cup powdered sugar
- 1 teaspoon vanilla extract
- ¼ teaspoon salt
- ¼ cup mini chocolate chips
- 2 tablespoons chopped pecans (optional)
- 20 wonton wrappers
- ¼ cup filtered water

Directions:
1. Preheat the air fryer to 370°F.
2. In a large bowl, use a hand mixer to combine the cream cheese with the powdered sugar, vanilla, and salt. Fold in the chocolate chips and pecans. Set aside.
3. Lay the wonton wrappers out on a flat, smooth surface and place a bowl with the filtered water next to them.
4. Use a teaspoon to evenly divide the cream cheese mixture among the 20 wonton wrappers, placing the batter in the center of the wontons.
5. Wet the tip of your index finger, and gently moisten the outer edges of the wrapper. Then fold each wrapper until it creates a secure pocket.
6. Liberally spray the air fryer basket with olive oil mist.
7. Place the wontons into the basket, and cook for 5 to 8 minutes. When the outer edges begin to brown, remove the wontons from the air fryer basket. Repeat cooking with remaining wontons.
8. Serve warm.

Fall Caramelized Apples

Servings: 2
Cooking Time: 25 Minutes

Ingredients:
- 2 apples, sliced
- 1 ½ tsp brown sugar
- ¼ tsp cinnamon
- ¼ tsp nutmeg
- ¼ tsp salt
- 1 tsp lemon zest

Directions:
1. Preheat air fryer to 390°F. Set the apples upright in a baking pan. Add 2 tbsp of water to the bottom to keep the apples moist. Sprinkle the tops with sugar, lemon zest, cinnamon, and nutmeg. Lightly sprinkle the halves with salt and the tops with oil. Bake for 20 minutes or until the apples are tender and golden on top. Enjoy.

Peanut Butter S'mores

Servings:10
Cooking Time: 1 Minute

Ingredients:

• 10 Graham crackers (full, double-square cookies as they come out of the package)
• 5 tablespoons Natural-style creamy or crunchy peanut butter
• ½ cup Milk chocolate chips
• 10 Standard-size marshmallows (not minis and not jumbo campfire ones)

Directions:

1. Preheat the air fryer to 350°F .
2. Break the graham crackers in half widthwise at the marked place, so the rectangle is now in two squares. Set half of the squares flat side up on your work surface. Spread each with about 1½ teaspoons peanut butter, then set 10 to 12 chocolate chips point side up into the peanut butter on each, pressing gently so the chips stick.
3. Flatten a marshmallow between your clean, dry hands and set it atop the chips. Do the same with the remaining marshmallows on the other coated graham crackers. Do not set the other half of the graham crackers on top of these coated graham crackers.
4. When the machine is at temperature, set the treats graham cracker side down in a single layer in the basket. They may touch, but even a fraction of an inch between them will provide better air flow. Air-fry undisturbed for 45 seconds.
5. Use a nonstick-safe spatula to transfer the topped graham crackers to a wire rack. Set the other graham cracker squares flat side down over the marshmallows. Cool for a couple of minutes before serving.

Coconut Crusted Bananas With Pineapple Sauce

Servings: 4
Cooking Time: 5 Minutes

Ingredients:

• Pineapple Sauce
• 1½ cups puréed fresh pineapple
• 2 tablespoons sugar
• juice of 1 lemon
• ¼ teaspoon ground cinnamon
• 3 firm bananas
• ¼ cup sweetened condensed milk
• 1¼ cups shredded coconut
• ⅓ cup crushed graham crackers (crumbs)*
• vegetable or canola oil, in a spray bottle
• vanilla frozen yogurt or ice cream

Directions:

1. Make the pineapple sauce by combining the pineapple, sugar, lemon juice and cinnamon in a saucepan. Simmer the mixture on the stovetop for 20 minutes, and then set it aside.
2. Slice the bananas diagonally into ½-inch thick slices and place them in a bowl. Pour the sweetened condensed milk into the bowl and toss the bananas gently to coat. Combine the coconut and graham cracker crumbs together in a shallow dish. Remove the banana slices from the condensed milk and let any excess milk drip off. Dip the banana slices in the coconut and crumb mixture to coat both sides. Spray the coated slices with oil.
3. Preheat the air fryer to 400°F.
4. Grease the bottom of the air fryer basket with a little oil. Air-fry the bananas in batches at 400°F for 5 minutes, turning them over halfway through the cooking time. Air-fry until the bananas are golden brown on both sides.
5. Serve warm over vanilla frozen yogurt with some of the pineapple sauce spooned over top.

Chocolate Rum Brownies

Servings: 6
Cooking Time: 30 Minutes + Cooling Time

Ingredients:

• ½ cup butter, melted
• 1 cup white sugar
• 1 tsp dark rum
• 2 eggs
• ½ cup flour
• 1/3 cup cocoa powder
• ¼ tsp baking powder
• Pinch of salt

Directions:

1. Preheat air fryer to 350°F. Whisk the melted butter, eggs, and dark rum in a mixing bowl until slightly fluffy and all ingredients are thoroughly combined. Place the flour, sugar, cocoa, salt,

and baking powder in a separate bowl and stir to combine. Gradually pour the dry ingredients into the wet ingredients, stirring continuously until thoroughly blended and there are no lumps in the batter. Spoon the batter into a greased cake pan. Put the pan in the frying basket and Bake for 20 minutes until a toothpick comes out dry and clean. Let cool for several minutes. Cut and serve. Enjoy!

Bananas Foster Bread Pudding

Servings: 4
Cooking Time: 25 Minutes

Ingredients:
- ½ cup brown sugar
- 3 eggs
- ¾ cup half and half
- 1 teaspoon pure vanilla extract
- 6 cups cubed Kings Hawaiian bread (½-inch cubes), ½ pound
- 2 bananas, sliced
- 1 cup caramel sauce, plus more for serving

Directions:
1. Preheat the air fryer to 350°F.
2. Combine the brown sugar, eggs, half and half and vanilla extract in a large bowl, whisking until the sugar has dissolved and the mixture is smooth. Stir in the cubed bread and toss to coat all the cubes evenly. Let the bread sit for 10 minutes to absorb the liquid.
3. Mix the sliced bananas and caramel sauce together in a separate bowl.
4. Fill the bottom of 4 (8-ounce) greased ramekins with half the bread cubes. Divide the caramel and bananas between the ramekins, spooning them on top of the bread cubes. Top with the remaining bread cubes and wrap each ramekin with aluminum foil, tenting the foil at the top to leave some room for the bread to puff up during the cooking process.
5. Air-fry two bread puddings at a time for 25 minutes. Let the puddings cool a little and serve warm with additional caramel sauce drizzled on top. A scoop of vanilla ice cream would be nice too and in keeping with our Bananas Foster theme!

White Chocolate Cranberry Blondies

Servings: 6
Cooking Time: 18 Minutes

Ingredients:
- ⅓ cup butter
- ½ cup sugar
- 1 teaspoon vanilla extract
- 1 large egg
- 1 cup all-purpose flour
- ½ teaspoon baking powder
- ⅛ teaspoon salt
- ¼ cup dried cranberries
- ¼ cup white chocolate chips

Directions:
1. Preheat the air fryer to 320°F.
2. In a large bowl, cream the butter with the sugar and vanilla extract. Whisk in the egg and set aside.
3. In a separate bowl, mix the flour with the baking powder and salt. Then gently mix the dry ingredients into the wet. Fold in the cranberries and chocolate chips.
4. Liberally spray an oven-safe 7-inch spring-form pan with olive oil and pour the batter into the pan.
5. Cook for 17 minutes or until a toothpick inserted in the center comes out clean.
6. Remove and let cool 5 minutes before serving.

Choco-granola Bars With Cranberries

Servings: 6
Cooking Time: 20 Minutes

Ingredients:
- 2 tbsp dark chocolate chunks
- 2 cups quick oats
- 2 tbsp dried cranberries
- 3 tbsp shredded coconut
- ½ cup maple syrup
- 1 tsp ground cinnamon
- ⅛ tsp salt
- 2 tbsp smooth peanut butter

Directions:
1. Preheat air fryer to 360°F. Stir together all

the ingredients in a bowl until well combined. Press the oat mixture into a parchment-lined baking pan in a single layer. Put the pan into the frying basket and Bake for 15 minutes. Remove the pan from the fryer, and lift the granola cake out of the pan using the edges of the parchment paper. Leave to cool for 5 minutes. Serve sliced and enjoy!.

Cinnamon Tortilla Crisps

Servings: 4
Cooking Time: 8 Minutes

Ingredients:
- 1 tortilla
- 2 tsp muscovado sugar
- ½ tsp cinnamon

Directions:
1. Preheat air fryer to 350°F. Slice the tortilla into 8 triangles like a pizza. Put the slices on a plate and spray both sides with oil. Sprinkle muscovado sugar and cinnamon on top, then lightly spray the tops with oil. Place in the frying basket in a single layer. Air Fry for 5-6 minutes or until they are light brown. Enjoy warm.

Coconut Cream Roll-ups

Servings: 4
Cooking Time: 20 Minutes

Ingredients:
- ½ cup cream cheese, softened
- 1 cup fresh raspberries
- ¼ cup brown sugar
- ¼ cup coconut cream
- 1 egg
- 1 tsp corn starch
- 6 spring roll wrappers

Directions:
1. Preheat air fryer to 350°F. Add the cream cheese, brown sugar, coconut cream, cornstarch, and egg to a bowl and whisk until all ingredients are completely mixed and fluffy, thick and stiff. Spoon even amounts of the creamy filling into each spring roll wrapper, then top each dollop of filling with several raspberries. Roll up the wraps around the creamy raspberry filling, and seal the seams with a few dabs of water.
2. Place each roll on the foil-lined frying basket,

seams facing down. Bake for 10 minutes, flipping them once until golden brown and perfect on the outside, while the raspberries and cream filling will have cooked together in a glorious fusion. Remove with tongs and serve hot or cold. Serve and enjoy!

Fried Banana S'mores

Servings: 4
Cooking Time: 6 Minutes

Ingredients:
- 4 bananas
- 3 tablespoons mini semi-sweet chocolate chips
- 3 tablespoons mini peanut butter chips
- 3 tablespoons mini marshmallows
- 3 tablespoons graham cracker cereal

Directions:
1. Preheat the air fryer to 400°F.
2. Slice into the un-peeled bananas lengthwise along the inside of the curve, but do not slice through the bottom of the peel. Open the banana slightly to form a pocket.
3. Fill each pocket with chocolate chips, peanut butter chips and marshmallows. Poke the graham cracker cereal into the filling.
4. Place the bananas in the air fryer basket, resting them on the side of the basket and each other to keep them upright with the filling facing up. Air-fry for 6 minutes, or until the bananas are soft to the touch, the peels have blackened and the chocolate and marshmallows have melted and toasted.
5. Let them cool for a couple of minutes and then simply serve with a spoon to scoop out the filling.

Mixed Berry Pie

Servings: 4
Cooking Time: 25 Minutes

Ingredients:
- 2/3 cup blackberries, cut into thirds
- ¼ cup sugar
- 2 tbsp cornstarch
- ¼ tsp vanilla extract
- ¼ tsp peppermint extract
- ½ tsp lemon zest
- 1 cup sliced strawberries

- 1 cup raspberries
- 1 refrigerated piecrust
- 1 large egg

Directions:

1. Mix the sugar, cornstarch, vanilla, peppermint extract, and lemon zest in a bowl. Toss in all berries gently until combined. Pour into a greased dish. On a clean workspace, lay out the dough and cut into a 7-inch diameter round. Cover the baking dish with the round and crimp the edges. With a knife, cut 4 slits in the top to vent.

2. Beat 1 egg and 1 tbsp of water to make an egg wash. Brush the egg wash over the crust. Preheat air fryer to 350°F. Put the baking dish into the frying basket. Bake for 15 minutes or until the crust is golden and the berries are bubbling through the vents. Remove from the air fryer and let cool for 15 minutes. Serve warm.

Nutty Cookies

Servings: 6
Cooking Time: 25 Minutes

Ingredients:

- ¼ cup pistachios
- ¼ cup evaporated cane sugar
- ¼ cup raw almonds
- ½ cup almond flour
- 1 tsp pure vanilla extract
- 1 egg white

Directions:

1. Preheat air fryer to 375°F. Add ¼ cup of pistachios and almonds into a food processor. Pulse until they resemble crumbles. Roughly chop the rest of the pistachios with a sharp knife. Combine all ingredients in a large bowl until completely incorporated. Form 6 equally-sized balls and transfer to the parchment-lined frying basket. Allow for 1 inch between each portion. Bake for 7 minutes. Cool on a wire rack for 5 minutes. Serve and enjoy.

Cherry Cheesecake Rolls

Servings: 6
Cooking Time: 30 Minutes

Ingredients:

- 1 can crescent rolls

- 4 oz cream cheese
- 1 tbsp cherry preserves
- 1/3 cup sliced fresh cherries

Directions:

1. Roll out the dough into a large rectangle on a flat work surface. Cut the dough into 12 rectangles by cutting 3 cuts across and 2 cuts down. In a microwave-safe bowl, soften cream cheese for 15 seconds. Stir together with cherry preserves. Mound 2 tsp of the cherries-cheese mix on each piece of dough. Carefully spread the mixture but not on the edges. Top with 2 tsp of cherries each. Roll each triangle to make a cylinder.

2. Preheat air fryer to 350°F. Place the first batch of the rolls in the greased air fryer. Spray the rolls with cooking oil and Bake for 8 minutes. Let cool in the air fryer for 2-3 minutes before removing. Serve.

Cherry Hand Pies

Servings: 8
Cooking Time: 8 Minutes

Ingredients:

- 4 cups frozen or canned pitted tart cherries (if using canned, drain and pat dry)
- 2 teaspoons lemon juice
- ½ cup sugar
- ¼ cup cornstarch
- 1 teaspoon vanilla extract
- 1 Basic Pie Dough (see the preceding recipe) or store-bought pie dough

Directions:

1. In a medium saucepan, place the cherries and lemon juice and cook over medium heat for 10 minutes, or until the cherries begin to break down.

2. In a small bowl, stir together the sugar and cornstarch. Pour the sugar mixture into the cherries, stirring constantly. Cook the cherry mixture over low heat for 2 to 3 minutes, or until thickened. Remove from the heat and stir in the vanilla extract. Allow the cherry mixture to cool to room temperature, about 30 minutes.

3. Meanwhile, bring the pie dough to room temperature. Divide the dough into 8 equal pieces. Roll out the dough to ¼-inch thickness in circles. Place ¼ cup filling in the center of each rolled dough. Fold the dough to create a half-circle.

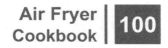

Using a fork, press around the edges to seal the hand pies. Pierce the top of the pie with a fork for steam release while cooking. Continue until 8 hand pies are formed.

4. Preheat the air fryer to 350°F.

5. Place a single layer of hand pies in the air fryer basket and spray with cooking spray. Cook for 8 to 10 minutes or until golden brown and cooked through.

Date Oat Cookies

Servings: 6
Cooking Time: 20 Minutes

Ingredients:
- ¼ cup butter, softened
- 2 ½ tbsp milk
- ½ cup sugar
- ½ tsp vanilla extract
- ½ tsp lemon zest
- ½ tsp ground cinnamon
- 3/4 cup flour
- ¼ tsp salt
- ¾ cup rolled oats
- ¼ tsp baking soda
- ¼ tsp baking powder
- 2 tbsp dates, chopped

Directions:
1. Use an electric beater to whip the butter until fluffy. Add the milk, sugar, lemon zest, and vanilla. Stir until well combined. Add the cinnamon, flour, salt, oats, baking soda, and baking powder in a separate bowl and stir. Add the dry mix to the wet mix and stir with a wooden spoon. Pour in the dates.

2. Preheat air fryer to 350°F. Drop tablespoonfuls of the batter onto a greased baking pan, leaving room in between each. Bake for 6 minutes or until light brown. Make all the cookies at once, or save the batter in the fridge for later. Let them cool and enjoy!

Pear And Almond Biscotti Crumble

Servings: 6
Cooking Time: 65 Minutes

Ingredients:
- 7-inch cake pan or ceramic dish
- 3 pears, peeled, cored and sliced
- ½ cup brown sugar
- ¼ teaspoon ground ginger
- 1 teaspoon ground cinnamon
- ⅛ teaspoon ground nutmeg
- 2 tablespoons cornstarch
- 1¼ cups (4 to 5) almond biscotti, coarsely crushed
- ¼ cup all-purpose flour
- ¼ cup sliced almonds
- ¼ cup butter, melted

Directions:
1. Combine the pears, brown sugar, ginger, cinnamon, nutmeg and cornstarch in a bowl. Toss to combine and then pour the pear mixture into a greased 7-inch cake pan or ceramic dish.

2. Combine the crushed biscotti, flour, almonds and melted butter in a medium bowl. Toss with a fork until the mixture resembles large crumbles. Sprinkle the biscotti crumble over the pears and cover the pan with aluminum foil.

3. Preheat the air fryer to 350°F.

4. Air-fry at 350°F for 60 minutes. Remove the aluminum foil and air-fry for an additional 5 minutes to brown the crumble layer.

5. Serve warm.

Mango Cobbler With Raspberries

Servings: 4
Cooking Time: 30 Minutes

Ingredients:
- 1 ½ cups chopped mango
- 1 cup raspberries
- 1 tbsp brown sugar
- 2 tsp cornstarch
- 1 tsp lemon juice
- 2 tbsp sunflower oil
- 1 tbsp maple syrup
- 1 tsp vanilla
- ½ cup rolled oats
- 1/3 cup flour
- 3 tbsp coconut sugar
- 1 tsp cinnamon
- ¼ tsp nutmeg
- ⅛ tsp salt

Directions:
1. Place the mango, raspberries, brown sugar, cornstarch, and lemon juice in a baking pan. Stir with a rubber spatula until combined. Set aside.

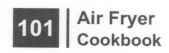

2. In a separate bowl, add the oil, maple syrup, and vanilla and stir well. Toss in the oats, flour, coconut sugar, cinnamon, nutmeg, and salt. Stir until combined. Sprinkle evenly over the mango-raspberry filling. Preheat air fryer to 320°F. Bake for 20 minutes or until the topping is crispy and golden. Enjoy warm.

Vegan Brownie Bites

Servings: 10
Cooking Time: 8 Minutes

Ingredients:
- ⅔ cup walnuts
- ⅓ cup all-purpose flour
- ¼ cup dark cocoa powder
- ⅓ cup cane sugar
- ¼ teaspoon salt
- 2 tablespoons vegetable oil
- 1 teaspoon pure vanilla extract
- 1 tablespoon almond milk
- 1 tablespoon powdered sugar

Directions:
1. Preheat the air fryer to 350°F.
2. To a blender or food processor fitted with a metal blade, add the walnuts, flour, cocoa powder, sugar, and salt. Pulse until smooth, about 30 seconds. Add in the oil, vanilla, and milk and pulse until a dough is formed.
3. Remove the dough and place in a bowl. Form into 10 equal-size bites.
4. Liberally spray the metal trivet in the air fryer basket with olive oil mist. Place the brownie bites into the basket and cook for 8 minutes, or until the outer edges begin to slightly crack.
5. Remove the basket from the air fryer and let cool. Sprinkle the brownie bites with powdered sugar and serve.

Maple Cinnamon Cheesecake

Servings: 4
Cooking Time: 12 Minutes

Ingredients:
- 6 sheets of cinnamon graham crackers
- 2 tablespoons butter
- 8 ounces Neufchâtel cream cheese
- 3 tablespoons pure maple syrup
- 1 large egg
- ½ teaspoon ground cinnamon
- ¼ teaspoon salt

Directions:
1. Preheat the air fryer to 350°F.
2. Place the graham crackers in a food processor and process until crushed into a flour. Mix with the butter and press into a mini air-fryer-safe pan lined at the bottom with parchment paper. Place in the air fryer and cook for 4 minutes.
3. In a large bowl, place the cream cheese and maple syrup. Use a hand mixer or stand mixer and beat together until smooth. Add in the egg, cinnamon, and salt and mix on medium speed until combined.
4. Remove the graham cracker crust from the air fryer and pour the batter into the pan.
5. Place the pan back in the air fryer, adjusting the temperature to 315°F. Cook for 18 minutes. Carefully remove when cooking completes. The top should be lightly browned and firm.
6. Keep the cheesecake in the pan and place in the refrigerator for 3 or more hours to firm up before serving.

Nutty Banana Bread

Servings: 6
Cooking Time: 30 Minutes

Ingredients:
- 2 bananas
- 2 tbsp ground flaxseed
- ¼ cup milk
- 1 tbsp apple cider vinegar
- 1 tbsp vanilla extract
- ½ tsp ground cinnamon
- 2 tbsp honey
- ½ cup oat flour
- ½ tsp baking soda
- 3 tbsp butter

Directions:
1. Preheat air fryer to 320°F. Using a fork, mash the bananas until chunky. Mix in flaxseed, milk, apple vinegar, vanilla extract, cinnamon, and honey. Finally, toss in oat flour and baking soda until smooth but still chunky. Divide the batter between 6 cupcake molds. Top with one and a half teaspoons of butter each and swirl it a little. Bake for 18 minutes until golden brown and puffy. Let cool completely before serving.

Vanilla Butter Cake

Servings: 6
Cooking Time: 20-24 Minutes

Ingredients:
- ¾ cup plus 1 tablespoon All-purpose flour
- 1 teaspoon Baking powder
- ¼ teaspoon Table salt
- 8 tablespoons (½ cup/1 stick) Butter, at room temperature
- ½ cup Granulated white sugar
- 2 Large egg(s)
- 2 tablespoons Whole or low-fat milk (not fat-free)
- ¾ teaspoon Vanilla extract
- Baking spray (see here)

Directions:
1. Preheat the air fryer to 325°F (or 330°F, if that's the closest setting).
2. Mix the flour, baking powder, and salt in a small bowl until well combined.
3. Using an electric hand mixer at medium speed, beat the butter and sugar in a medium bowl until creamy and smooth, about 3 minutes, occasionally scraping down the inside of the bowl.
4. Beat in the egg or eggs, as well as the white or a yolk as necessary. Beat in the milk and vanilla until smooth. Turn off the beaters and add the flour mixture. Beat at low speed until thick and smooth.
5. Use the baking spray to generously coat the inside of a 6-inch round cake pan for a small batch, a 7-inch round cake pan for a medium batch, or an 8-inch round cake pan for a large batch. Scrape and spread the batter into the pan, smoothing the batter out to an even layer.
6. Set the pan in the basket and air-fry undisturbed for 20 minutes for a 6-inch layer, 22 minutes for a 7-inch layer, or 24 minutes for an 8-inch layer, or until a toothpick or cake tester inserted into the center of the cake comes out clean. Start checking it at the 15-minute mark to know where you are.
7. Use hot pads or silicone baking mitts to transfer the cake pan to a wire rack. Cool for 5 minutes. To unmold, set a cutting board over the baking pan and invert both the board and the pan. Lift the still-warm pan off the cake layer.

Set the wire rack on top of the cake layer and invert all of it with the cutting board so that the cake layer is now right side up on the wire rack. Remove the cutting board and continue cooling the cake for at least 10 minutes or to room temperature, about 30 minutes, before slicing into wedges.

Baked Caramelized Peaches

Servings: 6
Cooking Time: 25 Minutes

Ingredients:
- 3 pitted peaches, halved
- 2 tbsp brown sugar
- 1 cup heavy cream
- 1 tsp vanilla extract
- ¼ tsp ground cinnamon
- 1 cup fresh blueberries

Directions:
1. Preheat air fryer to 380°F. Lay the peaches in the frying basket with the cut side up, then top them with brown sugar. Bake for 7-11 minutes, allowing the peaches to brown around the edges. In a mixing bowl, whisk heavy cream, vanilla, and cinnamon until stiff peaks form. Fold the peaches into a plate. Spoon the cream mixture into the peach cups, top with blueberries, and serve.

Date: _____

MY SHOPPING LIST

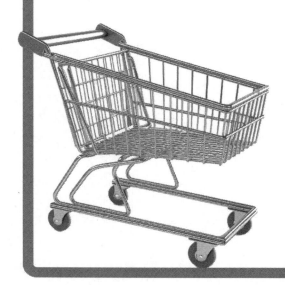

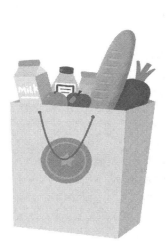

APPENDIX A: Measurement Conversions

BASIC KITCHEN CONVERSIONS & EQUIVALENTS

DRY MEASUREMENTS CONVERSION CHART

3 TEASPOONS = 1 TABLESPOON = 1/16 CUP

6 TEASPOONS = 2 TABLESPOONS = 1/8 CUP

12 TEASPOONS = 4 TABLESPOONS = 1/4 CUP

24 TEASPOONS = 8 TABLESPOONS = 1/2 CUP

36 TEASPOONS = 12 TABLESPOONS = 3/4 CUP

48 TEASPOONS = 16 TABLESPOONS = 1 CUP

METRIC TO US COOKING CONVERSIONS

OVEN TEMPERATURES

120 °C = 250 °F

160 °C = 320 °F

180° C = 350 °F

205 °C = 400 °F

220 °C = 425 °F

LIQUID MEASUREMENTS CONVERSION CHART

8 FLUID OUNCES = 1 CUP = 1/2 PINT = 1/4 QUART

16 FLUID OUNCES = 2 CUPS = 1 PINT = 1/2 QUART

32 FLUID OUNCES = 4 CUPS = 2 PINTS = 1 QUART
 = 1/4 GALLON

128 FLUID OUNCES = 16 CUPS = 8 PINTS = 4 QUARTS = 1 GALLON

BAKING IN GRAMS

1 CUP FLOUR = 140 GRAMS

1 CUP SUGAR = 150 GRAMS

1 CUP POWDERED SUGAR = 160 GRAMS

1 CUP HEAVY CREAM = 235 GRAMS

VOLUME

1 MILLILITER = 1/5 TEASPOON

5 ML = 1 TEASPOON

15 ML = 1 TABLESPOON

240 ML = 1 CUP OR 8 FLUID OUNCES

1 LITER = 34 FL. OUNCES

US TO METRIC COOKING CONVERSIONS

1/5 TSP = 1 ML

1 TSP = 5 ML

1 TBSP = 15 ML

1 FL OUNCE = 30 ML

1 CUP = 237 ML

1 PINT (2 CUPS) = 473 ML

1 QUART (4 CUPS) = .95 LITER

1 GALLON (16 CUPS) = 3.8 LITERS

1 OZ = 28 GRAMS

1 POUND = 454 GRAMS

BUTTER

1 CUP BUTTER = 2 STICKS = 8 OUNCES = 230 GRAMS = 8 TABLESPOONS

WHAT DOES 1 CUP EQUAL

1 CUP = 8 FLUID OUNCES

1 CUP = 16 TABLESPOONS

1 CUP = 48 TEASPOONS

1 CUP = 1/2 PINT

1 CUP = 1/4 QUART

1 CUP = 1/16 GALLON

1 CUP = 240 ML

WEIGHT

1 GRAM = .035 OUNCES

100 GRAMS = 3.5 OUNCES

500 GRAMS = 1.1 POUNDS

1 KILOGRAM = 35 OUNCES

BAKING PAN CONVERSIONS

1 CUP ALL-PURPOSE FLOUR = 4.5 OZ

1 CUP ROLLED OATS = 3 OZ 1 LARGE EGG = 1.7 OZ

1 CUP BUTTER = 8 OZ 1 CUP MILK = 8 OZ

1 CUP HEAVY CREAM = 8.4 OZ

1 CUP GRANULATED SUGAR = 7.1 OZ

1 CUP PACKED BROWN SUGAR = 7.75 OZ

1 CUP VEGETABLE OIL = 7.7 OZ

1 CUP UNSIFTED POWDERED SUGAR = 4.4 OZ

BAKING PAN CONVERSIONS

9-INCH ROUND CAKE PAN = 12 CUPS

10-INCH TUBE PAN = 16 CUPS

11-INCH BUNDT PAN = 12 CUPS

9-INCH SPRINGFORM PAN = 10 CUPS

9 X 5 INCH LOAF PAN = 8 CUPS

9-INCH SQUARE PAN = 8 CUPS

Appendix B : Recipes Index

A

Air-fried Turkey Breast With Cherry Glaze 48
Almond Green Beans 51
Apple Crisp 96
Apple Dumplings 95
Apple-cinnamon-walnut Muffins 12
Asian Glazed Meatballs 72
Asian-style Flank Steak 38
Asparagus, Mushroom And Cheese Soufflés 68
Authentic Sausage Kartoffel Salad 32
Avocado Toast With Lemony Shrimp 20
Avocado Toasts With Poached Eggs 13

B

Bacon Candy 27
Baked Caramelized Peaches 103
Baked Eggs 10
Baked Shishito Peppers 55
Balsamic Marinated Rib Eye Steak With Balsamic Fried Cipollini Onions 36
Bananas Foster Bread Pudding 98
Basil Crab Cakes With Fresh Salad 86
Bbq Chips 26
Beef Short Ribs 31
Berbere Eggplant Dip 64
Best-ever Roast Beef Sandwiches 72
Better-than-chinese-take-out Sesame Beef 37
Bite-sized Blooming Onions 63
Black Bean Veggie Burgers 73
Blueberry French Toast Sticks 9
Blueberry Muffins 10
Breakfast Frittata 11
Brie-currant & Bacon Spread 18
Buffalo Wings 19
Buttermilk Biscuits 16
Buttermilk-fried Drumsticks 41
Buttery Rolls 52
Buttery Stuffed Tomatoes 54

C

Cajun Flounder Fillets 85
Caprese-style Sandwiches 65
Catfish Nuggets 87
Charred Radicchio Salad 55
Cheddar Bean Taquitos 67
Cheddar-bean Flautas 64
Cheese & Bacon Pasta Bake 56
Cheese & Crab Stuffed Mushrooms 87
Cheese Straws 21
Cheeseburger Slider Pockets 24
Cheesy Chicken Tenders 41
Cheesy Spinach Dip 20
Cherry Cheesecake Rolls 100
Cherry Hand Pies 100
Chicago-style Turkey Meatballs 42
Chicano Rice Bowls 64
Chicken Apple Brie Melt 80
Chicken Club Sandwiches 75
Chicken Gyros 76
Chicken Nuggets 44
Chicken Saltimbocca Sandwiches 79
Chicken Souvlaki Gyros 47
Chicken Spiedies 80
Chicken Wellington 48
Chicken Wings Al Ajillo 41
Chili Cheese Dogs 83
Chinese-style Lamb Chops 34
Chinese-style Potstickers 23
Chipotle Chicken Drumsticks 44
Choco-granola Bars With Cranberries 98
Chocolate Rum Brownies 97
Cinnamon Tortilla Crisps 99
Cinnamon-stick Kofta Skewers 29
Citrus Baked Scallops 90
Coconut Cream Roll-ups 99
Coconut Crusted Bananas With Pineapple Sauce 97
Coconut-shrimp Po' Boys 91
Coffee Cake 14
Collard Green & Cod Packets 93
Corn Dog Bites 27
Country Wings 19
Cowboy Rib Eye Steak 30
Crab Rangoon 23
Crabmeat-stuffed Flounder 85
Crispy Cauliflower Puffs 51
Crispy Samosa Rolls 11
Crispy Spiced Chickpeas 23
Crunchy Clam Strips 93
Crunchy Falafel Balls 78
Crunchy Pickle Chips 18

D

Date Oat Cookies 101
Delicious Juicy Pork Meatballs 31
Dijon Artichoke Hearts 52
Dijon Thyme Burgers 82
Double Cheese-broccoli Tots 58

E

Easy Bread Pudding 95
Easy Turkey Meatballs 43
Easy-peasy Shrimp 91
Eggless Mung Bean Tart 11
Eggplant Parmesan Subs 82

F

Falafel 62
Fall Caramelized Apples 96
Favourite Fried Chicken Wings 46
Fennel & Chicken Ratatouille 46
Feta & Shrimp Pita 93
Fish Sticks For Kids 92
Friday Night Cheeseburgers 35
Fried Banana S'mores 99
Fried Cannoli Wontons 96
Fried Dill Pickle Chips 19
Fried Pb&j 15
Fried Rice With Curried Tofu 69

G

Garlic Bread Knots 12
Golden Breaded Mushrooms 66
Golden Fried Tofu 65
Green Bean & Baby Potato Mix 68
Green Beans 59
Green Egg Quiche 14
Green Onion Pancakes 8
Grits Again 58
Ground Beef Calzones 36

H

Hazelnut Chicken Salad With Strawberries 42
Herbed Baby Red Potato Hasselback 53
Holliday Lobster Salad 89
Home-style Fish Sticks 90
Homemade Chips Ahoy 95

Homemade Pretzel Bites 22
Honey-mustard Roasted Cabbage 55
Hot Cauliflower Bites 18
Hungarian Pork Burgers 29

I

Inside Out Cheeseburgers 77
Inside-out Cheeseburgers 75
Intense Buffalo Chicken Wings 46
Italian Stuffed Bell Peppers 63

J

Jalapeño Poppers 21

K

Kale & Lentils With Crispy
Onions 61
Korean-style Lamb Shoulder
Chops 35

L

Lamb Burgers 74
Lemon Pork Escalopes 31
Lemony Tuna Steaks 91
Lentil Fritters 70
Lorraine Egg Cups 11

M

Maewoon Chicken Legs 40
Mango Cobbler With
Raspberries 101
Maple Cinnamon Cheesecake 102
Maple-peach And Apple Oatmeal 10
Mashed Potato Taquitos With Hot
Sauce 8
Meatless Kimchi Bowls 63
Meaty Omelet 9
Mediterranean Salmon Burgers 88
Mexican Cheeseburgers 77
Mexican Turkey Meatloaves 45
Mixed Berry Pie 99
Morning Loaded Potato Skins 9
Morning Potato Cakes 9
Moroccan Cauliflower 53
Mushroom-rice Stuffed Bell
Peppers 62

N

Nordic Salmon Quiche 12
Nutty Banana Bread 102
Nutty Cookies 100
Nutty Shrimp With Amaretto
Glaze 92

O

Orange-glazed Carrots 25

P

Panko-crusted Zucchini Fries 54
Paprika Onion Blossom 26
Parmesan Crackers 26
Parmesan Portobello Mushroom
Caps 62
Parsley Egg Scramble With Cottage
Cheese 13
Parsnip Fries With Romesco
Sauce 59
Peachy Pork Chops 34
Peanut Butter S'mores 97
Pear And Almond Biscotti
Crumble 101
Peppered Steak Bites 33
Peppery Tilapia Roulade 88
Perfect Broccoli 57
Perfect Broccolini 55
Perfect Burgers 81
Philly Cheesesteak Sandwiches 77
Pickle Brined Fried Chicken 49
Pine Nut Eggplant Dip 70
Pizza Dough 13
Pizza Portobello Mushrooms 67
Poblano Bake 40
Pork Chops 37
Provolone Stuffed Meatballs 76

Q

Quinoa Burgers With Feta Cheese
And Dill 66

R

Reuben Sandwiches 83
Rich Salmon Burgers With Broccoli
Slaw 89
Rich Turkey Burgers 42
Roasted Brussels Sprouts 56
Roasted Thyme Asparagus 51
Roasted Vegetable Frittata 15
Roasted Vegetable Stromboli 61

S

Salmon Burgers 78
Salmon Puttanesca En Papillotte
With Zucchini 88
Satay Chicken Skewers 43
Sausage And Pepper Heros 81
Sea Salt Radishes 53
Sesame Orange Tofu With Snow
Peas 65
Sesame-crusted Tuna Steaks 90
Shrimp Egg Rolls 22
Shrimp Patties 90
Simple Roasted Sweet Potatoes 53
Simple Salsa Chicken Thighs 41
Simple Zucchini Ribbons 56

Sirloin Steak Flatbread 34
Skirt Steak With Horseradish
Cream 30
Southern Okra Chips 56
Spanish Fried Baby Squid 24
Spiced Parsnip Chips 25
Spicy Black Bean Turkey Burgers With
Cumin-avocado Spread 47
Spicy Hoisin Bbq Pork Chops 32
Spring Vegetable Omelet 14
Sriracha Short Ribs 33
Steakhouse Burgers With Red Onion
Compote 30
Street Corn 58
Stuffed Pork Chops 33
Stuffed Shrimp Wrapped In
Bacon 92
Sunday Chicken Skewers 44
Sweet & Spicy Swordfish Kebabs 86
Sweet And Sour Pork 36
Sweet And Spicy Pumpkin Scones 16
Sweet Plantain Chips 20
Sweet Roasted Carrots 69

T

Taco Pie With Meatballs 35
Teriyaki Chicken Drumsticks 45
Tex-mex Fish Tacos 87
Thai-style Pork Sliders 73
Thanksgiving Turkey Sandwiches 74
Tomato Candy 57
Tuna Patties With Dill Sauce 85
Turkey Burgers 45
Turkey Tenderloin With A Lemon
Touch 43
Turkey-hummus Wraps 42
Tuscan Salmon 89

V

Vanilla Butter Cake 103
Vegan Brownie Bites 102
Vegan French Toast 67
Vegetarian Shepherd's Pie 68
Vegetarian Stuffed Bell Peppers 69
Veggie Chips 25
Veggie Fritters 57
Viking Toast 8

W

White Bean Veggie Burgers 79
White Chocolate Cranberry
Blondies 98
Wiener Schnitzel 29
Wrapped Shrimp Bites 18

Z

Zesty London Broil 32

Made in United States
Orlando, FL
18 November 2024

54085104R00061